He's
LOOKIN'
at You, Kid!

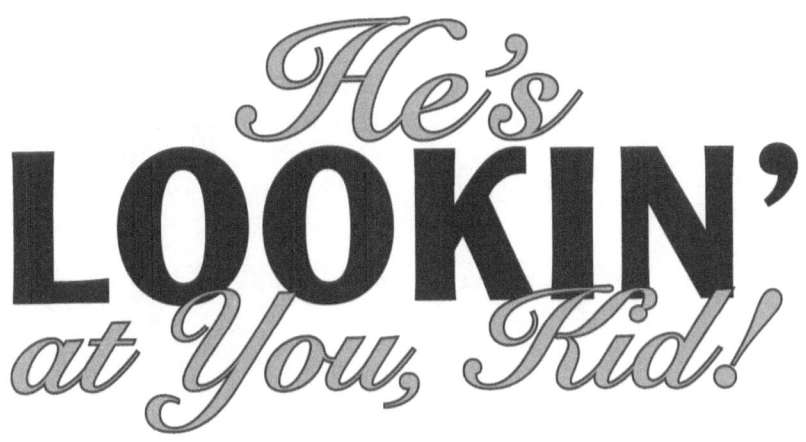

He's LOOKIN' at You, Kid!

A story of hope and faith that God can get you through anything you face in life because He is faithful to watch over His children!

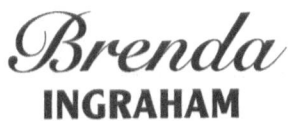

Brenda INGRAHAM

iUniverse, Inc.
New York   Bloomington

"He's Lookin' At You, Kid!"

iUniverse books may be ordered through booksellers or by contacting:

iUniverse
1663 Liberty Drive
Bloomington, IN 47403
www.iuniverse.com
1-800-Authors (1-800-288-4677)

ISBN: 978-0-595-48116-3 (pbk)
ISBN: 978-0-595-60216-2 (ebk)

Printed in the United States of America
Cover: Design by Vertical Communications, LLC.
Photos by Tony Frantz Photography
Sunrise background photo by Robyn MacKenzie/iStock

iUniverse rev. date: 1/21/09

Acknowledgements

When friends and associates encouraged me to write a book about what God had done in my life and my personal battles through six long years with breast cancer, I literally laughed out loud, saying, "I am not a writer!" which is true. I have come to learn more about how God truly operates when He has a plan. More specifically, when He wants a story told. God will take your spoken word about what you cannot do and have you do that very thing. He knows that you know, it is not you completing the task, but it is His Holy Spirit working through you.

1 Corinthians 1:27- But God chose the foolish things of the world to shame the wise; God chose the weak things of the world to shame the strong.

How can someone who has never written before, complete a book within three months? When I was told I needed to deal more with the pain, I asked, "How do I accomplish that?" I prayed that entire day and told God I had no clue how to put on paper the deep pain from the wounds to my soul. How do you possibly relate how painful the situation really was? I sat at my computer and, in four hours to be precise, God wrote the chapter, "In The Midst Of The Pain." Therefore, I want to give my biggest THANKS to my Heavenly Father who authored this book through me. I am humbled to be used to present the truth of God's Word as it relates in our daily life. *Thank you for loving me, caring for me, watching over every aspect of my life, and giving me hope and a purpose!*

I would also like to thank my beautiful daughters, Christina and Stephanie, for encouraging me to stay on course, which is hard for someone with ADD to do. Your love and support means the world to me. I thank my dearest sisters in the Lord, Sandy Souza and Rhonda White, who have been my support and spiritual 'cheerleaders.' You have pioneered the way for others to believe they have a story to tell. May God use this book to inspire others as your books have done.

I thank Drs.' Oscar and Sharron Underwood for speaking into my life the HOPE I needed to believe there was truly a future ahead of me. I thank Eric Schoening of Vertical Communications for bringing God's eyes to life on the book cover and Tony Frantz for capturing the joy and beauty of God's love through his photography! You are both truly gifted. I thank Cathy Dee for her patience in editing. You have been such a blessing!

I thank Rico Marable of Light Life E-media for producing my CD, "Refined Hope" and encouraging me to put this book into audio form. What a divine revelation for those who would rather listen than to read. To my readers (and listeners!), I thank you for understanding as I open my heart to you and try to translate into words the magnitude of God's love that He has for each of us, His children.

Foreword

One Sunday morning, while still sleepy and only semi-conscious, I found myself thinking about my life and what God had gotten me through. Once I fully woke up, those thoughts were still there. I felt as if I should put them down on paper, so I went to my computer and spent several hours typing away. I couldn't seem to stop. I continued, and after one week, amazingly found that I had typed the entire basis for this book. Was God speaking to me? Was God inspiring and directing me?

In this book, I write often about God *speaking* to me, or God *telling* me what to do in my life. I truly believe it was God who woke me up that Sunday morning and that He continued to move through me as I wrote.

I believe God desires to, and can, speak to each and everyone about the great love and plan He has for them. The problem comes with our *listening*. As in any relationship, there needs to be communication. Prayer is our part of the communication process, but how does God speak to us?

First and foremost, God speaks to us through His Word, The Holy Bible. I view the Bible as God's love letters to us. I've experienced periods when a Scripture I've read hundreds of times seems to jump off the page to get my attention. It never fails to be a Scripture that speaks directly to something that is going on in my life and is exactly what I need to hear.

God spoke to Elijah in *1Kings 19:11-13 - The LORD said, "Go out and stand on the mountain in the presence of the LORD, for the LORD is about to pass by."*

Then a great and powerful wind tore the mountains apart and shattered the rocks before the LORD, but the LORD was not in the wind. After the wind there was an earthquake, but the LORD was not in the earthquake. After the earthquake came a fire, but the LORD was not in the fire. And after the fire came **a gentle whisper**. *When Elijah heard it, he pulled his cloak over his face and went out and stood at the mouth of the cave. Then a voice said to him, "What are you doing here, Elijah?"*

As this Scripture says, His voice is a "gentle whisper." There have only been two occasions when I actually heard a voice, a very soft and calming male voice. Was the voice audible or was it in my head? I'm not sure, but I do know that I heard it and I followed its direction.

When I asked God about going to the doctor in Nashville to see if I could develop my falsetto, I didn't hear a voice, but I did hear Him in my heart-- literally. It was a very long dialogue that I sensed in my chest and resonated in my thought process. Every time I have *sensed* Him speaking, there has been a peace, calmness, and a *knowing* in my Spirit that it was God.

I get the same sensation when I sense that someone is staring at me. I don't know for sure someone is staring until I look around and confirm it. It's that same *knowing* in my Spirit when God speaks. The Word says the sheep know the Shepherd's voice. As His children, we *can* recognize His voice and hear Him say, "I'm lookin' at you, kid!"

It is clear through the twists and turns in Brenda's life that God had His eyes on her. But what is even more revealing is that she had her eyes on Him. Her book shares most intimate details of her journey and is a must read. We all have challenges; however, Brenda's faith is a great testimony of how to walk, talk and see during those challenges.

-- Sandy Souza, Author
Embracing loss...a message of hope

Truly "He's Looking At You, Kid!" will be a great blessing to millions for generations to come! Brenda is a living testimony that no matter what you go through (for God's Glory); where God is taking you TO will be greater than what you go through. Expect to be reassured that we have a Heavenly Father who neither slumbers nor sleeps, but is watching over us through sunshine and rain (Isaiah 45). Brenda's PASSION for life has now been birthed out of her Pain to encourage the world - Enjoy!"

-- Rhonda A. White, CNHP and Author "The INNERgizer"
Stop Going In The Tent Without Any Intent!   Eagle Inspirations
"Clean The Clutter Before I Tell Your Mother!"   Dare 2 Declare!

Brenda's story reminds us that not only is God's eye always upon us, but His hands are always at work in our story. If you need encouragement to keep trusting in God's heart, soak up Brenda's story of redemption; her life is a testimony to God's willingness to turn ashes to beauty, to bring hope from despair. Learn from Brenda's story and let God lead you into the life He sees for you.

-- Tim Hallman; Pastor
Anchor Community Church

Psalm 121

I lift up my eyes to the hills—
where does my help come from?
My help comes from the LORD,
the Maker of heaven and earth.

He will not let your foot slip—
He who watches over you will not slumber.

Indeed, He who watches over Israel
will neither slumber nor sleep.

The LORD watches over you—
the LORD is your shade at your right hand.

The sun will not harm you by day,
nor the moon by night.

The LORD will keep you from all harm—
He will watch over your life.

The LORD will watch over your coming and going
both now and forevermore.

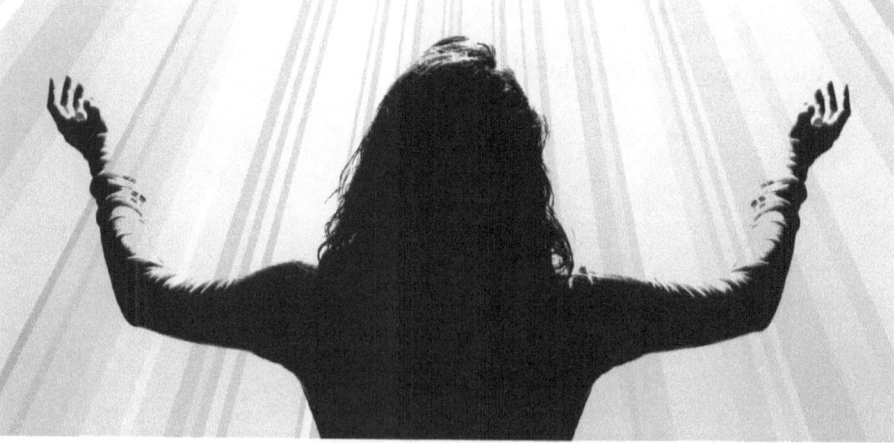

Contents

Chapter One

Family Matters

I have always sensed a presence in my life, a presence that made me feel safe, secure, happy, and at peace. I knew God was watching over my family. I also knew He was watching over me. There is assurance that, as a loving heavenly Father, "He's lookin' at you, kid!"

Our Father loves you so much that He can't take His eyes off of you because He cares and wants only the best for you. He has a good plan for your life. We are told many times in the Bible that He will never leave us nor forsake us (*Deuteronomy 31:6 and 8, Joshua 1:5*). What a promise to know that the God who created this universe loves us that much.

As a young child, I looked at the world through eyes of amazement and awe. Everything was good and people were kind and loving, but that was in the '50s, when life was simple and easy. I was so innocent and thought things were exactly as they seemed. It's funny how I thought "life time warranty" meant my lifetime, and I thought the countryside would change when I crossed the state line. Living life would open my eyes to the truth of reality. Life is complicated and rarely turns out the way we imagined or thought it would.

My mother met my father, who was five years older, at a lake park. They both were only children. Their first meeting was not your typical "boy meets

1

girl and falls head over heels in love;" but rather, boy almost drowns young girl when he encourages her to ride on the zip-line trellis into the water. He didn't realize she couldn't swim and ended up saving her life.

My mother had a beautiful operatic voice and was offered a scholarship to college. What a rare opportunity for a young woman in that era, but my father gave her the ultimatum of either going to college or spending her life with him. She chose my father and was married at sixteen. I loved to hear my mother when she used her singing gift in church. I have often thought how differently her life might have been if she had not been given that ultimatum. I think my father felt he might lose my mother if she went to college because she was a beautiful and personable young woman. However, I believe by doing this, my father didn't allow my mother to reach her full potential to be who God created her to be. Being aware of this truth in my parent's life has shaped how I view relationships and why I feel mutual respect and compromise is important in making a relationship stronger.

I was the baby of five children; my only sister, seven when I was born, was the oldest. My father worked hard as a lab technician for Dupont to provide for his family, but was rarely there to provide the emotional support we really needed. When he was home, he was reading the paper, working in the garage or visiting with a neighbor. I don't recall my father sitting down with me just to ask how school was going or to inquire about what was happening in my life. I am not sure he knew how to have a meaningful conversation. I would classify him as an absentee father even though he was home

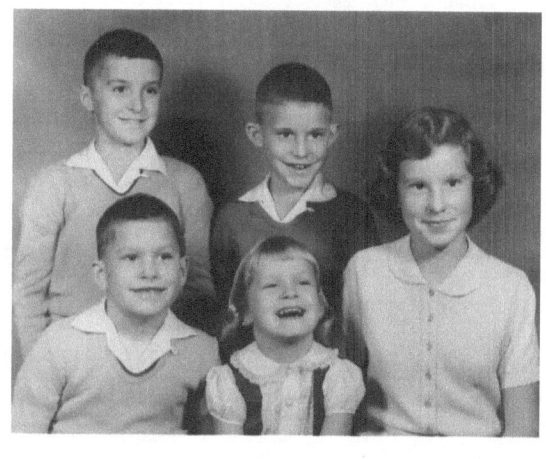

physically every day. I believe my mother became the dominant parent because my father relinquished the control to her, which was common in the '50s, because the man's role was to be the financial provider while the woman took care of the home.

My father was adopted and very faithful to his adoptive mother and grandmother. This tie was so strong that it created issues in my parent's marriage, affecting our entire family. Growing up, my life was filled with arguing. The good news is that with our arguing, the issue was dealt with then put behind us so we could start over fresh. I know there are a lot of families that are quite the opposite. Instead of arguing or talking loudly, as I like to say, they rarely raise their voice to each other; but they also do not talk about the important issues that are happening in their family. They skirt around the fact that there is a huge elephant in the room. Having lived with both types of families, I believe it's essential to find balance. I have yet to see a family that is not dysfunctional in one form or another. After years of counseling, I have come to realize how important it is to deal with issues in love and try to find win-win solutions for the problems.

Every situation we face and every person that comes into our lives helps to mold us into the person we become. We can choose the outcome by how we decide to allow situations and people to affect us. When I married, I learned that not all families argued. There was actually another way of dealing with people. On the other hand, huge issues that dealt with emotions and even life and death were not talked about.

Today, with a divorce behind us, I see that my daughters look at marriage differently. One thinks it is a fantasy to have a wonderful marriage while the other is determined to never divorce. As you read about my life, you will learn how wild and crazy I was; and yet it was living the nightclub lifestyle that has made me the determined, passionate, and devout Christian that I am today. Everything that happens to us molds our thought process, but we determine by our choice which direction we will take.

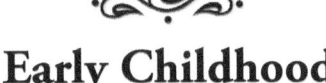

Early Childhood

Growing up the baby of five children, I had to be loud and outgoing to be noticed. At least that was my excuse! The common belief is that the baby of the family is spoiled. I disagree. It took a lot of effort for me to be heard. The only advantage I saw in being the youngest was that my parents were much more lenient with me as a teenager than with my sister. I didn't have the strict rules and responsibilities she had as the oldest. It seemed that my parents were more fearful with their first child; but by the time I came along, it was smooth sailing. I have always loved my life and the people that were in it. My view of life has always been that the glass is half full. I never met a stranger and I saw everyone as good. That is one positive aspect of having a Type A, sanguine personality. Even from an early age, my perspective has always been positive.

Perspective On Life

Author Unknown

One day, the father of a very wealthy family took his son on a trip to the country with the express purpose of showing him how poor people live. They spent a couple of days and nights on the farm of what would be considered a very poor family.

On their return from their trip, the father asked his son, "How was the trip?" "It was great, Dad." "Did you see how poor people live?" the father asked. "Oh yeah," said the son. "So, tell me, what did you learn from the trip?" asked the father.

The son answered, "I saw that we have one dog and they have four. We have a pool that reaches to the middle of our garden and they have a creek that has no end. We have imported lanterns in our garden and they have the stars at night. Our patio reaches to the front yard and they have the whole horizon. We have a small piece of land to live on and they have fields that go beyond our sight. We have servants who serve us, but they serve others. We buy our food, but they grow theirs. We have walls around our property to protect us, they have friends to protect them." The boy's father was speechless. Then his son added, "Thanks Dad for showing me how poor we are."

Isn't perspective a wonderful thing? Makes you wonder what would happen if we all gave thanks for everything we have, instead of worrying about what we don't have.

At the age of five, I had several accidents that challenged my natural optimistic attitude. But my positive resolve would continue on throughout my life and the hardships I would face as an adult. God promises us protection.

Isaiah 43:2-3 - When you pass through the waters, I will be with you; and when you pass through the rivers, they will not sweep over you. When you walk through the fire, you will not be burned; the flames will not set you ablaze. For I am the LORD, your God, the Holy One of Israel, your Savior.

I can't remember anything from before I was five. A counselor once told me that something must have happened to traumatize me, but I believe it was because of all my falls on the back of my head. I remember my mother telling me about a time when I was two years old. They found me climbing a ladder to the roof but I fell off, hitting the back of my head. My mom said I fell on the back of my head many times but was never seriously injured. I guess that is one advantage of being hardheaded!

I love to get dizzy on spinning rides at the amusement park. One accident happened when I was twirling around in a circle trying to make myself dizzy. I fell on a pile of rocks and cut a gash on my right wrist. We didn't go to the doctor for stitches because it was not bad enough to pay the price for the doctor bill. The scar is very noticeable and the enemy would use that scar to convince me I could commit suicide later in life because I didn't remember it hurting very much.

My grandmother had a very mean dog named Tip that liked no one except my grandmother. When I was asked to feed Tip, he seemed friendly toward me for the first time, wagging his tail and following me since I had the food. When I sat the food down, he became very mean again, growling as I tried to pet him. No one told me you shouldn't pet a dog while he is eating. Suddenly Tip bit me in the face. I have a scar as a reminder to never pet a dog at suppertime. I like to think the scar looks like a dimple since it's located where a dimple would be.

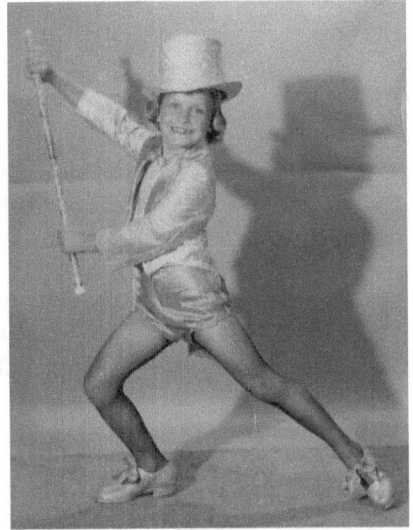

Another accident happened while I practiced tap dancing with two of my friends. We decided to put a trick into the routine. They would swing me from the porch while holding onto my hands and feet. I cracked the back of my head on the edge of the concrete porch. The neighbor across the street heard my head hit and came to help. I was not taken to the doctor this time either because you didn't go to the doctor for something minor in those days.

The worst scar I would receive that year was from disobeying one of my mother's rules. She had told me on numerous occasions not to ride on the back of a bike, but I didn't listen. When my friend hit a bump, my foot went into the sprocket chain and cut a gash in my right heel so deep you could see the bone. I remember my mother carrying me into the doctor's office with the blood from my heel all over us. We were both screaming. They wrapped me in a sheet to hold me still while they injected the needle to numb the area for preparation of the seventeen stitches needed to close the gash. Even though I had a hard year at age five, I still maintained my optimistic attitude.

The world we lived in during the '50s was so trusting. That same year my mother took all five of us grocery shopping. There was a mechanical pony ride in the entrance to the store. I begged my mother to let me stay and ride the pony while she shopped. I stayed on that pony for a very long time talking to people as they entered the store. I wondered what was taking my mother so long. To my surprise, I saw her coming in the front entrance of the store as I sat on the pony. She had gone all the way home before she discovered I was missing. I am not sure how we missed seeing each other when she left. I know that God's watchful eye of protection was on me as I was left alone in that store. It is tough to think what could have happened, but life then was much safer than today.

·᠅ᡣᡍᡪᡤ᠄·

School Days

My school-age memories are very, very happy ones. I loved the social aspect of school. I felt like I belonged. I would walk through the hallways with great pride thinking, "This is my school and I love it." I struggled academically and got C's in comprehension and conduct. I found out as an adult that I am ADD. This helped me to understand why I could not sit still, why it was so hard to focus for any length of time, why I would get in trouble with the teacher because I was talking, and why I hated to read. I still struggle with some of these issues but have learned to cope.

I have always been a firm believer in treating everyone as an equal, loving each person for who they are and granting them dignity and respect. I didn't like cliques because they excluded people, and those involved acted as though they were better than others. If we could live by the Golden Rule, _Matthew 7:12 -Do to others what you would have them do to you,_ the world would be a much better place.

I was fortunate to be the cheerleading mascot for the Junior Varsity football and basketball teams when I was a third grader. With modesty ruling the day for the older girls, I was the only one allowed to do cartwheels and flips.   I remained on the cheerleading squad throughout high school and was the only girl to ever be named football and basketball homecoming queen the same year.

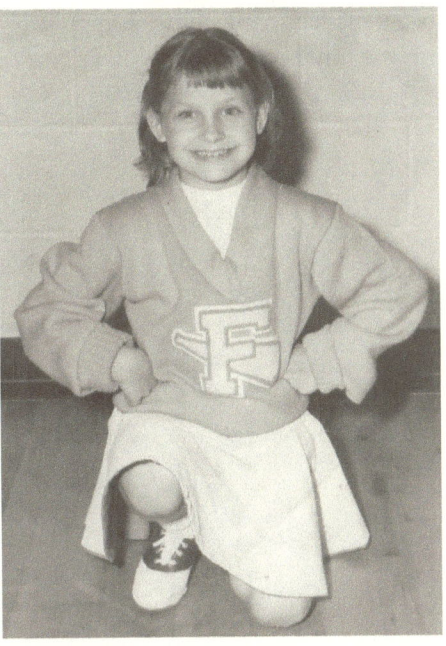

At my twenty-fifth class reunion, I was given the best compliment a person could receive. I was feeling very insecure and unhappy because of my pending divorce when a friend came over to me and said, "Are your ears burning because our entire table has been talking about you?" I asked if the comments were bad, but was assured they were positive. "We were talking about how you were one of the only people in our entire class who treated everyone just the same. It didn't matter if they were jocks, geeks, rich or poor." That one comment made a huge difference in my life. It made me see that even in my pain, I was not the person I had been portrayed to be in my marriage. It gave me a confidence to know it is okay to be who God created me to be.

I entered and won the Miss Fairdale beauty pageant in 1971. I couldn't believe they allowed me to win after I had told the judges during my interview that I had no plans to attend college. I was young, naive, and didn't know this pageant was a scholarship pageant. As winner of the Miss Fairdale pageant, I was automatically entered into the Miss Kentucky pageant. This would be the last year for the Miss Kentucky contest to be televised. I had to beg my father to attend just one night of the pageant. He loved to attend the athletic events for my brothers but had no desire to come to this type of venue. After much coaxing, he came for the final night. I was honored to be named in the top 10 and have my parents there to witness it.

Up to this point in my life, everything was really good. Most everyone I knew was a Christian and attended church. People were kind, courteous, and would actually smile at one another and say "Hello." You could leave your doors unlocked and not be afraid. We lived in America, a Christian nation that was founded on Christian principles. That would never have been challenged in those days as it is today. Being raised in church was the richest inheritance I could have ever been given.

Chapter Two

Spiritual Truths

My life experience has proven to me that true beauty comes from within. I have never been nor will I ever be a raving beauty. How many of us are truly physically beautiful? Most of us are pretty ordinary looking. Sure we try to make ourselves look better by putting on makeup, fixing our hair, and dressing in the best fashion, but most of us are not over-the-top gorgeous. I've heard that only two percent of the world's population is truly beautiful.

I love the anti-smoking advertisement showing a young girl with her face split in two. The right side was her normal face while her left side showed what she looked like inside from the effects of smoking. I wish life could be that simple. If only our faces could reveal what we really are on the inside. There would be no more Ted Bundy's, the charming and articulate serial killer who confessed to murdering thirty women between 1974 and 1978. We wouldn't be fooled or harmed by a deceptive person's outer beauty.

Growing up in a church environment and what I learned there played a huge roll in my belief system. As human beings, we are made up of body, mind and spirit. Because we are spiritual beings, we are influenced either by God to do good or satan (I refuse to capitalize his name) to do evil. Which influence do you allow to rule your spirit? Do you operate out of love or hate, gentleness or anger?

Proverbs 10:12 - Hatred stirs up dissension but love covers over all wrong.

Galatians 5:20-23 - Idolatry and witchcraft; hatred, discord, jealousy, fits of rage, selfish ambition, dissensions, factions and envy; drunkenness, orgies, and the like. I warn you, as I did before, that those who live like this will not inherit the kingdom of God. **But the fruit of the Spirit is love, joy, peace, patience, kindness, goodness, faithfulness, gentleness and self-control.**

Are you aware that satan was the most beautiful angel in heaven? His real name was Lucifer. He was second only to God and was in charge of music and worship. His pride and thirst for power and control became his downfall. When he decided he should be in charge instead of God, he led a revolt and persuaded a third of the angelic beings to follow him. Can you imagine the deception and lies it would take to convince an angel to turn against the God of the universe who created them?

Those same spirits were thrown out of heaven and now reign throughout the earth. They are referred to as the power of the air (*Ephesians 2:2*). Satan is the prince of this world (*John 12:31*) and the "god" of this world (*2 Corinthians 4:4*). The world is under satan's control (*1 John 5:19*), but God is the victor and we are victorious through Him.

1 John 4:4 KJV - Greater is He (God) that is in you than he (satan) that is in the world.

The appearance of satan is not how he is often portrayed--with horns and a pitchfork. He works his plan through people and loves to appear beautiful and good so we won't be afraid of him, then he will be able to weave us into his web of destruction. His goal is to take as many souls as possible to hell with him. Author Frank Peretti has a phenomenal way of showing the spiritual warfare we face through his fictional books. I highly recommend them, as they will enlighten you to the depths of spiritual warfare.

2 Corinthians 11:14 - For satan himself masquerades as an angel of light.

Matthew 12:43 - 45 - When an evil spirit comes out of a man, it goes through arid places seeking rest and does not find it. Then it says, 'I will return to the house I left.' When it arrives, it finds the house unoccupied, swept clean and put in order. Then it goes and takes with it seven other spirits more wicked than itself, and they go in and live there. And the final condition of that man is worse than the first. That is how it will be with this wicked generation.

We must remember that our battle is not with a person, but the spiritual force that is working through that person. God fights for us and is our protection against those spiritual forces.

Ephesians 6:11 –12 - Put on the full armor of God so that you can take your stand against the devil's schemes. For our struggle is not against flesh and blood, but against the rulers, against the authorities, against the powers of this dark world and against the spiritual forces of evil in the heavenly realms.

Isaiah 54:17 NKJV - No weapon forged against you will prosper.

Joshua 23:10 - One of you routs a thousand because the Lord, your God fights for you just as He promised.

Does Evil Exist?
Author Unknown

Does evil exist? The university professor challenged his students with this question. Did God create everything that exists? A student bravely replied, "Yes, he did!"

"God created everything?" The professor asked. "Yes sir", the student replied. The professor answered, "If God created everything, then God created evil since evil exists, and according to the principal that our works define who we are then God is evil."

The student became quiet before such an answer. The professor was quite pleased with himself and boasted to the students that he had proven once more that the Christian faith was a myth. Another student raised his hand and said, "Can I ask you a question, professor?" "Of course", replied the professor. The student stood up and asked, "Professor, does cold exist?" "What kind of question is this? Of course it exists. Have you never been cold?" The students snickered at the young man's question.

The young man replied, "In fact sir, cold does not exist. According to the laws of physics, what we consider cold is in reality the absence of heat. Every body or object is susceptible to study when it has or transmits energy, and heat is what makes a body or matter have or transmit energy. Absolute zero (- 460 degrees F) is the total absence of heat; all matter becomes inert and incapable of reaction in that temperature. Cold does not exist. We have created this word to describe how we feel if we have no heat.

The student continued. "Professor, does darkness exist?" The professor responded, "Of course it does." The student replied, "Once again you are wrong sir, darkness does not exist either. Darkness is in reality the absence of light. Light we can study, but not darkness. In fact, we can use Newton's prism to break white light into many colors and study the various wave lengths of each color. You cannot measure darkness. A simple ray of light can break into a world of darkness and illuminate it. How can you know how dark a certain space is? You measure the amount of light present. Isn't this correct? Darkness is a term used by man to describe what happens when there is no light present."

Finally the young man asked the professor. "Sir, does evil exist?" Now uncertain, the professor responded, "Of course, as I have already said. We see it every day. It is in the daily example of man's inhumanity to man. It is in the multitude of crime and violence everywhere in the world. These manifestations are nothing else but evil."

To this the student replied, "Evil does not exist sir, or at least it does not exist unto itself. *Evil is simply the absence of God*. It is just like darkness and cold, a word that man has created to describe the absence of God. God did not create evil. Evil is not like faith or love that exist, just as does light and heat. Evil is the result of what happens when man does not have God's love present in his heart. It's like the cold that comes when there is no heat or the darkness that comes when there is no light." The professor sat down.

The young man's name --- Albert Einstein

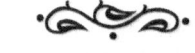

Allah Or Jesus?

This is a true story by author, Rick Mathes, a well-known leader in prison ministry. The event took place in the fall of 2003.

Last month I attended my annual training session that's required for maintaining my state prison security clearance. During the training session there was a presentation by three speakers representing the Roman Catholic, Protestant and Muslim faiths, who explained each of their belief systems.

I was particularly interested in what the Islamic Imam had to say. The Imam gave a great presentation of the basics of Islam, complete with a video. After the presentations, time was provided for questions and answers. When it was my turn, I directed my question to the Imam and asked: "Please, correct me if I'm wrong, but I understand that most Imams and clerics of Islam have declared a holy jihad [Holy war] against the infidels of the world. And, that by killing an infidel, which is a command to all Muslims, they are assured of a place in heaven. If that's the case, can you give me the definition of an infidel?"

There was no disagreement with my statements and, without hesitation, he replied, "Nonbelievers!" I responded, "So, let me make sure I have this straight. All followers of Allah have been commanded to kill everyone who is not of your faith so they can go to Heaven. Is that correct?" The expression on his face changed from one of authority and command to that of a little boy who had just gotten caught with his hand in the cookie jar. He sheepishly replied, "Yes." I then stated, "Well, sir, I have a real problem trying to imagine Pope John Paul commanding all Catholics to kill those of your faith or Dr. Stanley ordering Protestants to do the same in order to go to Heaven!"

The Imam was speechless. I continued, "I also have a problem with being your friend when you and your brother clerics are telling your followers to kill me. Let me ask you a question. *Would you rather have your Allah who tells you to kill me in order to go to Heaven or my Jesus who tells me to love you because I am going to Heaven and He wants you to be with me?*" You could have heard a pin drop as the Imam hung his head in shame.

As children of God, He gives us discernment through His Holy Spirit to have the ability to tell the difference between what is good and what is not. The deeper our relationship grows in the Lord, the more discernment He gives us to sense evil when it is presented to us. As we get into His Word, the Bible, we learn more about the spiritual battle and God's standard of what is right and what is wrong. He speaks to us through His still small voice (I Kings 19:12), directing us of the steps to take and guiding us through life for His good purpose.

I Kings 3:9 - So give your servant a discerning heart to govern your people and to distinguish between right and wrong.

James 4:7 - Resist the devil and he will flee from you. Come close to God and God will come close to you.

Proverbs 21:2 - A man's ways seem right to him, but the LORD weighs the heart.

I Chronicles 29:17 - I know, my God, that you test the heart and are pleased with integrity.

Jeremiah 17:10 - I, the Lord search the heart and examine the mind to reward a man according to his conduct according to what his deeds deserve.

Two Traveling Angels
Author Unknown

Two traveling angels stopped to spend the night in the home of a wealthy family. The family was rude and refused to let the angels stay in the mansion's guest room. Instead the angels were given a small space in the cold basement. As they made their bed on the hard floor, the older angel saw a hole in the wall and repaired it. When the younger angel asked why, the older angel replied, "Things aren't always what they seem."

The next night the pair came to rest at the house of a very poor, but very hospitable farmer and his wife. After sharing what little food they had, the couple let the angels sleep in their bed where they could have a good night's rest. When the sun came up the next morning, the angels found the farmer and his wife in tears. Their only cow, whose milk had been their sole income, lay dead in the field. The younger angel was infuriated and asked the older angel, "How could you have let this happen?"

The first man had everything, yet you helped him, she accused. The second family had little but was willing to share everything, and you let the cow die. "Things aren't always what they seem," the older angel replied. "When we stayed in the basement of the mansion, I noticed there was gold stored in that hole in the wall. Since the owner was so obsessed with greed and unwilling to share his good fortune, I sealed the wall so he would not find it. Then last night as we slept in the farmer's bed, the angel of death came for his wife. I gave him the cow instead. Things aren't always what they seem."

That is exactly what happens when things do not turn out the way we think they should. In the midst of my trials, I may question what God is doing. The answer may not be clear to me because things are not always as they seem. God's ways are higher and deeper than our human minds can imagine. *Isaiah 55:9 - "As the heavens are higher than the earth, so are my ways higher than your ways and my thoughts than your thoughts."* If we have faith, we just need to trust that every outcome can be used to our advantage. We may never know why, but we must continue to trust!

I thought my life was all about me and what I wanted; but as I get older I realize that I was created for His purpose, to share with others His love and His plan of salvation. I am not the harvester, the one actually bringing people into His kingdom; I am the seed sower, planting seeds of hope and faith that help people desire to get to know Him better.

Philippians 2:13 - It is God who works in you to will and to act according to His good purpose.

John 14:6 - Jesus answered, "I am the way and the truth and the life. No one comes to the Father except through me."

Acts 4:12 - Salvation is found in no one else, for there is no other name under heaven given to men by which we must be saved.

Psalms 62:1 - My soul finds rest in God alone; my salvation comes from Him.

Why Go To Church?
Author Unknown

A Churchgoer wrote a letter to the editor of a newspaper and complained that it made no sense to go to church every Sunday. "I've gone for 30 years now," he wrote, "and in that time I have heard something like 3,000 sermons. But for the life of me, I can't remember a single one of them. So, I think I'm wasting my time and the pastors are wasting theirs by giving sermons at all."

This started a real controversy in the "Letters to the Editor" column, much to the delight of the editor. It went on for weeks until someone wrote this clincher: "I've been married for 30 years now. In that time my wife has cooked some 32,000 meals. But, for the life of me, I cannot recall the entire menu for a single one of those meals. But I do know this ... they all nourished me and gave me the strength I needed to do my work. If my wife had not given me these meals, I would be physically dead today. Likewise, if I had not gone to church for nourishment, I would be spiritually dead today!"

When you are DOWN to nothing.... God is UP to something! Faith sees the invisible, believes the incredible and receives the impossible! Thank God for our physical and our spiritual nourishment!

I have heard it said many times that the church is full of hypocrites. I see the church as a hospital where hurting people come for healing. Each person is at a different stage of being ill, but all need help. We find strength through other believers. The church building is just that, a building. The actual church is the body of Christ made of believers that come to assemble themselves together in worshiping our Lord. The visible church has always been a mixture of spiritual and carnal believers, and unsaved persons.

I know many people who have been hurt by the church but you must remember it was the enemy using people in the church to wound you. His goal is to appear as an angel of light and to divide and conquer. We get lost easier when we are on our own. There is power as believers come together. In _Acts 2_ the power of the Holy Spirit came as they were in one accord. Fellowship, edification, and lifting each other up come when we are in communion with one another. When we are in fellowship, we become accountable for our actions. Accountability keeps us on track and headed in the right direction.

I Corinthians 3:16 - Don't you know that you yourselves are the temple of God and that God's Spirit lives in you?

Hebrews 10:24-25 - And let us consider how we may spur one another on toward love and good deeds. Let us not give up meeting together, as some are in the habit of doing, but let us encourage one another—and all the more as you see the Day approaching.

Acts 2:42-47 - They devoted themselves to the apostles' teaching and to the fellowship, to the breaking of bread and to prayer. Everyone was filled with awe, and many wonders and miraculous signs were done by the apostles. All the believers were together and had everything in common. Selling their possessions and goods, they gave to anyone as he had need. Every day they continued to meet together in the temple courts.

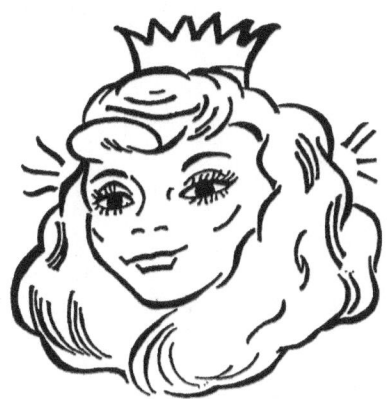

This sketch epitomizes what we look like on the inside with Christ as our Savior. Turn the book upside down to see what we look like without Christ in our life! GREAT example, don't you think?

Chapter Three

Nightclub Life

I grew up attending many Protestant denominations because my mother was a "church hopper." She was looking for a deeper walk with God. I went through the motions of baptism at ten years of age in a Baptist Church without full understanding of what baptism represented or meant. I had a life changing, 'born again' experience at thirteen in the Church of God.

During my marriage, we attended a Quaker Church; and after the divorce, my daughters and I grew spiritually in an Assembly of God Church. Now, we attend an interdenominational church. The bottom line is not which church you attend. It's about your relationship with Jesus Christ. I am not talking about religion. I'm talking about having a personal, intimate relationship with the Creator of the universe, the God, out of who brought the world into existence with His spoken word. It's possible to know Him intimately. He's not "the man upstairs," out of reach, but a loving heavenly Father that desires for His children to know Him.

I left the church when I started singing professionally in nightclubs at age eighteen. I should not have been in a nightclub because I was underage; but somehow, that was never an issue since I was a member of the band. My singing partner, Juanita, was the same age as I. We became fast friends and remain as close as sisters to this day.

I was very naïve when I started singing professionally so when dirty jokes were told during our breaks, I did not laugh because I didn't understand them. A waitress kept calling me "tree," saying, "Brenda, if your IQ was one point lower, you would be a tree." I understood what she meant--that I was stupid because I didn't get the dirty jokes. The enemy, satan, would use this comment to make me determined to understand everything and to never be naïve again.

This would be the hook to draw me into the web of the worldly, low standards; lying, cheating, smoking, drinking, drugs, sex…. a world of emptiness and loneliness. Oh yes, I made fabulous money, but at what cost? The money could not buy me the happiness, peace, joy and contentment I had known in my life before entering the nightclub scene. Living this lifestyle came at a very high price. The saying: *Sin takes you farther than you want to go, makes you stay longer than you want to stay, and costs you more than you want to pay,* was so very true in my life.

1 Corinthians 15:33 -*Do not be misled: "Bad company corrupts good character."* This is what happened to me. It's true that you become like the people you hang around. No matter how hard you try, you take on their characteristics. This is the reason parents are concerned with their children's friends. *Proverbs 20:11* - *Even a child is known by his actions, by whether his conduct is pure and right.* I was a Christian when I went into the nightclubs but I certainly was not when I came out.

The nightclub life seemed glamorous at first. I could not believe that I was making more money than my father. His money was used to provide for a family of seven. Over my four-year career, I sang with three different groups. My first concert was performed at the Toys for Tots fundraiser in Louisville, Kentucky with over 35,000 in attendance. Our group was featured in the front-page photograph the Courier Journal used to tell about the concert's huge success. I had the opportunity to "party" with the Wolfman Jack tour while they stayed at the Ramada Inn where we were performing in Louisville.

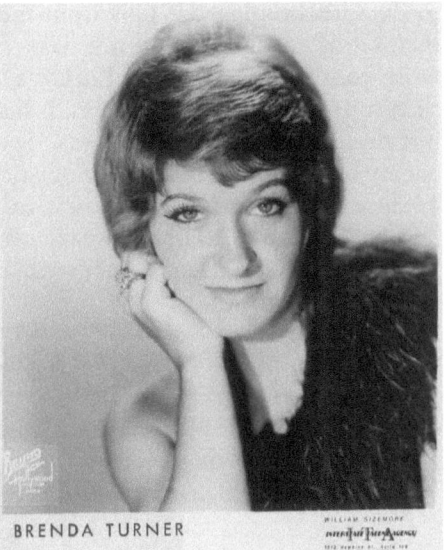

BRENDA TURNER

My big break came when Juanita and I were asked to sing with Ronnie Dove, who had six gold records in the 1960s. His notoriety was before my time, so I was not impressed as were fans that came to hear him sing. Juanita decided not to take the job, so I ended up going on my own. I would open the show with a song, be Ronnie's backup singer, and he would feature me during the show. People were trying to get to Ronnie through me, so I was lavished with gifts and special treatment. It didn't take long before I became self-centered, egotistical, and thought life revolved around me.

Contemplating Suicide

At the end of my fourth year in the nightclubs, I began to contemplate suicide very seriously; not just because of the immorality of my lifestyle, but also because of the person I had become. I hated myself because I knew it was not the real me. The Lord was convicting me of my sinful lifestyle and wooing me to come back to Him, but I did not know how to get back. There were no Christians in the nightclubs and I was no longer attending church, so my only way out seemed to be to end my life through suicide. The thoughts kept whirling through my head. No one was aware of my inner agony because I had learned how to put on a mask. To see me, you would have thought I was the happiest person in the world. No one could see the pain and self-hatred I had for the person I had become during those dark years of my life.

I had arranged to get some pills on three different occasions because just going to sleep seemed to be the easiest way to die, but the drugs never came through. Amazing, since the ability to score any type of drug you wanted was easy in the nightclubs. I didn't think that God might have had something to do with keeping the pills from me until I started contemplating a new method of suicide: slicing my wrist. As I looked at the scar on my right wrist from falling as a child, I heard a voice say, "That didn't hurt, you could slice your wrist and your pain and this turmoil will finally be over." I shake just thinking how desperate I was. Self-hatred is a huge weapon used by the enemy to bring us to the point of suicide, but God was 'lookin' out for me, because of His great love and concern. God had a different plan for my life. The enemy knows all of our weak areas and will take full advantage of them. The Word of God tells us exactly what satan desires to do to each of us.

John 10:10 NKJV - The thief does not come except to steal, and to kill, and to destroy. I (Jesus) have come that they may have life and that they may have it more abundantly.

1 Peter 5:8 - Be self-controlled and alert. Your enemy the devil prowls around like a roaring lion looking for someone to devour.

At that exact time of contemplating suicide, God intervened. The polyps I had on my vocal chords from misuse while cheerleading began to grow. Edema, which is a fluid swelling, started in my vocal chords and forced the need for surgery. I had surgery to correct the problem on March 17, 1975. My doctor told me to not talk for six weeks. Some people say the real miracle was that I really didn't talk for that period of time!

Coming Home

I moved back home with my parents, and started attending a new church, one of the Assembly of God. As soon as I walked through the doors, I could feel the sweet presence of God. I watched as people lifted their hands, closed their eyes and prayed out loud. I knew they had a personal relationship with the Lord that I did not yet have, but I longed for. I rededicated my life to God and finally felt the joy, peace, and contentment I had missed for all those years. God was so faithful to keep me from ending my life and bringing me back home into His presence. No amount of money can buy what God freely gives to those who love Him.

One of the greatest gifts of salvation, besides knowing where I will spend eternity, is knowing that all of the sins I had committed in my past were not only washed away by the blood Jesus shed for us on the cross, but were forgotten as well. Forgiving myself was the hardest part of the process. Even though I knew I had been forgiven, I couldn't seem to forget my past until God released me one Sunday evening at a church service. What I heard was a message straight from the throne of God. Why should I hold onto my past, when God clearly was not?

Psalm 103:12 - As far as the east is from the west, so far has He removed our transgressions from us.

Isaiah 43:25 -"I, even I, am He who blots out your transgressions for my own sake and remembers your sins no more."

Isaiah 1:18 - Though your sins are like scarlet, they shall be as white as snow.

Jeremiah 31:34 - I will forgive their wickedness, and will remember their sin no more.

2 Corinthians 5:17 NKJV - Therefore, if anyone is in Christ, he is a new creation; old things have passed away, behold all things have become new.

I was a completely new creation, just as Scripture says. I was grateful to put my past where it belonged -- **behind me**.

When I went for my checkup after the surgery, the doctor asked me to speak. I opened my mouth but all that came out was a hoarse, low, gravely noise. He told me that the surgery had been a success, but the healing process had not. My left vocal chord healed in three layers instead of a single smooth layer. The doctor felt horrible when he told me I would never sing again. I use to joke that I could be a trio all by myself, since I could hit three notes at the same time every time I tried to sing. Although my surgery was a failure to the doctor, I could see God's hand all over this situation.

The musical group I was with had released an album two weeks before my surgery. They told me they would wait as long as necessary for me to come back to the group. The inability to sing was my ticket out of the nightclub life. If I had been able to sing, I would have gone back into the nightclubs and probably met my death. God wanted to give me "life." He spared me from the inner torment I had experienced, and gave me a second chance.

Overcoming Addictions

When I came back to the Lord, all of my sins were forgiven, but there was one sin I could not stop -- my addiction to marijuana. On two occasions, one of those was when we partied with Wolfman Jack's group; I suffered from hallucinations while smoking marijuana. I found out later that the marijuana had been laced with LSD. In my mind, I was running down a long tunnel toward a light, but could never reach the light at the end. The light always stayed the same distance away from me. In the other hallucination, I was on the backside of a kaleidoscope and every time I tried to step through, someone would turn it. On both occasions, I cried out to God and told Him I would give Him my life if He would allow me to get back into my right mind. He did get me back into my right mind, but I did not keep my promise. I was still in the nightclubs, which made it easy to continue with my addiction.

After rededicating my life to the Lord, I would go to church, come home and roll a joint to enjoy in the privacy of my own home. After a month of trying to quit my addiction, I cried out to God. I confessed that I had tried to quit, but couldn't. I knew this was not a good witness for my Christian walk and that it was not good for my health to continue. I begged Him to take away the desire. He answered my prayer once again. I sensed the desire was gone and immediately took my "dime" bag of marijuana and flushed it down the toilet. I have never desired it since.

How many of us have our secret sins that happen in the privacy of our own homes? In our hearts we know it is not right but we don't know how to break the habit. I hear people say, "I'm a good person and haven't done anything really bad." Whose scale is being used to determine what is bad? We live in a world where there is clearly a battle between good and evil. The world's view has shifted so much that right seems wrong and wrong seems right. Jesus is the plumb line for measuring our goodness. He alone knows our heart.

Do you know what a plumb line is? A plumb line is a simple but accurate tool used for determining whether or not something is perfectly vertical i.e. upright. The Lord's plumb line shows how righteously people stand (righteous actually means upright) according to His Word.

Romans 3:23 - *For all have sinned and fall short of the glory of God.*

Romans 14:23 - *Everything that does not come from faith is sin.*

James 4:17 - *Anyone, then, who knows the good he ought to do and doesn't do it, sins.*

2 Chronicles 6:30 - *Forgive, and deal with each man according to all he does since You know his heart, for You alone know the hearts of men.*

Growing In The Lord

The first eighteen months after the throat surgery, I was in church every time the doors were open. I devoured the Word, the Bible, because I was so hungry for all that the Lord had for me. One morning, I woke up and found my speaking voice a little more clear. I remember telling God that I had misused the gift He had given me and I would use my voice only for His purpose if He chose to heal me—and He did. The healing was not instantaneous; it took quite a few months before it was complete.

I started singing with a trio named Sweet Charity. In the beginning of the healing process, there were times when I would try to sing a note and nothing, not a sound, would come out. As the tenor, it would not make or break anything if some of my notes did not come out just right. Our vocal chords are muscles that need to be strengthened like any other muscle. Singing with Sweet Charity helped to strengthen and continue the healing of my vocal chords. However, I would not get my full range. I had a two-and-a-half octave range prior to the surgery, but only a ten-note range afterwards. My falsetto, the Sandy Patti-type voice, was gone.

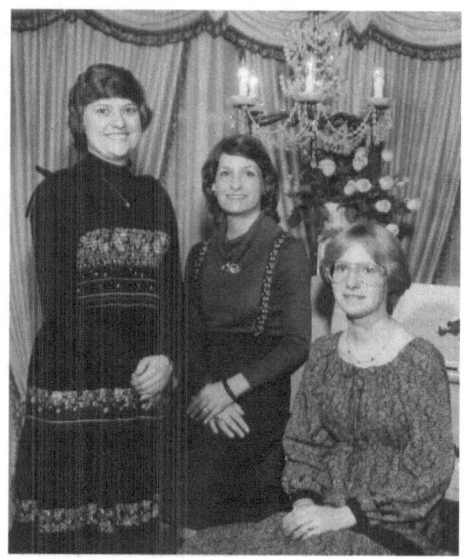

I was afraid to let anyone know that I only had a ten-note range because sometimes, we Christians can kill our own wounded. I was afraid that some well-intentioned soul would tell me there was a problem with my faith if I didn't get my entire range back. Finally, God released me from that fear of what other people thought and gave me two instructions He wanted me to now share:

1) *He does not want our ability. He wants our availability. If we make ourselves available, He will give us what we need to accomplish what He has for us to do.*

2) *Do not let the things you cannot do keep you from doing the things that you can.* Instead of looking at the two-and-a-half octave range I didn't have, I focused on the ten notes that I did have.

I am not a songwriter, but God certainly is. He gave me the song, *Available*, which was birthed from what He had told me. I put this song on my first CD titled, *Change*. It speaks about making ourselves available for Him to use. There are many songs I would love to sing but I don't have the range. I make sure the songs I do share have a powerful message of hope, encouragement, and God's love.

Music plays a crucial role in our society and can touch our soul in a way a sermon might not. In the Old Testament, musicians and singers were in front of the warriors leading the way into battle. When evil spirits tormented King Saul, the smooth music David would play on his harp would calm the King's spirit and help to bring peace to his soul.

Ministry

When I left the nightclub life, I started working a 'real' job in the Human Resources Department for a large bank in Louisville. Because I was 25 years old and not married, the girls in the department felt it was their duty to find me a man. The project started by seeing how many bachelors there were in the building around my age. They proceeded to pull the files of six single men so I could see their photos. The 'bets were on' as to who would be best suited for me. There were two men that came to the top of the list. I was taken on a tour of the building that just happened to allow me to meet the available single men. By the time I returned to my desk, I had a call requesting that I substitute for the bank's bowling team. The rest as they say, is history.

After I married, my husband was hired as Manager for a Credit Union, which required a move to Indiana. Word got out about my testimony and in 1981, I started "New Creation Ministries." The ministry was based on *2 Corinthians 5:17 NKJV - Therefore, if anyone is in Christ, he is a new creation; old things have passed away, behold all things have become new.* What an awesome promise! I had the wonderful opportunity to share in various churches and women's groups about God's healing power, God's mercy of sparing my life, and God's grace for a second chance on life. God's grace is *not getting* what I deserve because of my guilt and God's mercy is *getting* what I do not deserve, the freedom of guilt from my sin.

I felt that God wanted me to record a Christian tape of my favorite contemporary songs. I needed money for the recording so I asked God to provide it. He did just that, by allowing me to go into business selling promotional products. However, since balance has always been difficult for me and I am an "all or nothing" type of person, I became immersed with the business.

After a year of being consumed with the business and not with ministering, God spoke to me through a dream that the business was killing the ministry. In the dream, I was married to two men with no names, one, a blonde and the other, a brunette. We were married in the church and the church sanctioned our union. I loved them both, they loved me and they loved each other. Life was wonderful! One night we went to a theater to watch a play. Suddenly, the two were up on the stage. The blonde was waving a knife around the brunette's head, quoting Shakespeare. I knew the blonde was going to kill the brunette. At that moment, I realized that I did love the brunette more and that the blonde must have picked up on that. I stood up and screamed at the top of my lungs, "No don't," but before I could get the words out, the blonde slit the brunette's throat and ran away. I couldn't believe my "perfect" life had ended in ruins...the brunette, whom I truly loved was dead and the blonde was gone. While aimlessly walking the street, I thought that perhaps it really was a play, so I turned to go back to the theater.

I woke up from the dream at that moment. It was 4 a.m. and the emotions of the dream were deeply coursing through my body. The first words out of my mouth were, "I know this dream was from you Lord. What are you trying to show me?" Immediately, I knew the two men in the dream were symbolic and I was told, "the business is killing the ministry."

I told the Lord I would call the producer to start production on my CD project, but three days passed without following through. The next day I was given the scripture, *Ecclesiastes 5:5 - It is better to not make a vow then to make a vow and not fulfill it.* By this time, I knew I had been disobedient. I immediately called and started production. The tape titled, *Change*, was completed in 1993. Little did I know of the change that would take place the next year when my husband would file for divorce.

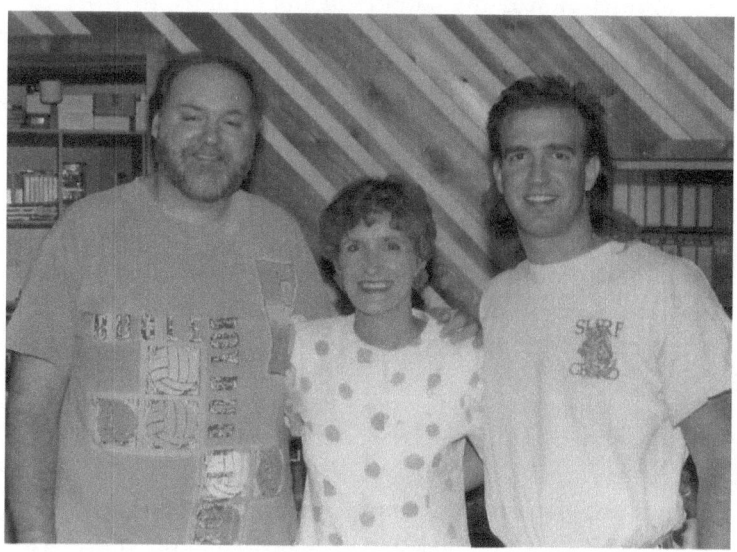

Darrell Powell & Greg Gilpin at Studio D Recording Studio

Chapter Four

Divorce

I never thought I would end up divorced. How could this possibly happen? We were a highly respected Christian couple working hard in our community and raising two beautiful daughters. All I can say, in retrospect, is that communication breakdown was one tool used by satan to end the dreams of living "until death do us part."

I have seen Christian couple after Christian couple torn apart because the enemy is actively working to break up the family, part of the body of Christ, through selfishness, pride, poor communication, extra-marital affairs, abuse, and power/control issues. Divorce is devastating to everyone involved. It is a wound that takes God's intervention to heal. I heard on a recent television program that the divorce rate for pastors is 52%. How very sad that the percentage of divorce in the church is that high.

Divide and conquer seems to be the method used by satan to shake the foundation of the faith as he works through people. It is amazing how after the divorce is final, those who were once your friends and family cease to have anything to do with you because they feel they have to take sides. This only adds to the pain of divorce and causes even more division. It's like cutting off the entire right side of your body and trying to function with what is left. One day you have a family; the next day you don't. Holidays are especially hard because they are reminders of the division. Things get even more painful and complicated when "step" parents and "step" siblings are introduced into the mix.

I know the divorce shook the foundation of my faith and what I believed to be the truth. I was totally crushed to the point of not being able to function. I didn't even make minimum wage for the first two years. I stopped singing because I had lost all of my joy and could not understand how God would allow this to happen. I did everything I knew to do scripturally to keep our marriage together. I would fast and pray for unity. I would bind the work of the enemy and loosen God's Holy Spirit (*Matthew 16:19*) to work in our marriage, but nothing helped.

It would take eight years for me to feel free from the pain of the divorce. Since the most attacks throughout the divorce were against my Type A, sanguine personality, it took four years in counseling to realize it was okay to be who God created me to be. It took just as long to understand that God will not go against a person's will. You cannot force someone to love you.

I've heard it said that the same thing that draws people to each other is inevitably the thing that ends up destroying the marriage. I found that to be true. I was loved for being an outgoing, fun-loving, and spontaneous woman. I loved him for being a responsible and hard-working man. In the end, I saw him as a workaholic who spent little time at home building a relationship with his family, and he saw me as a talkative, irresponsible woman who needed far too much attention. As John Gray so eloquently addresses the differences between men and women in his book, *Men Are From Mars, Women Are From Venus*, differences can be overcome with understanding of those differences; but the key is the desire to work at it.

The most important factor to any marriage must be that Jesus Christ is the foundation of the marriage. He is the building block on which the marriage must stand. As believers, we are instructed not to marry unbelievers.

2 Corinthians 6:14 - *Do not be yoked together with unbelievers. For what do righteousness and wickedness have in common? Or what fellowship can light have with darkness?*

At one of our Christian counseling sessions, my husband said the real problem in our marriage was that God was first in my life. I thought, "Well, how easy this is going to be to solve because when God is first in both of our lives, He's the bond that holds us together."

I kept waiting for the Christian counselor's response. When he did not acknowledge that it is crucial for God to be the center of a Christian marriage, I shared my feelings. I told my husband, "You've always been a 'good' guy. There is a Scripture that states, "to him who has been forgiven much, loves much" (*Luke 7:41- 47*). That's me. God took me out of a life of much sin and forgave me. I am that one who loves Him much. If you have a problem with my relationship with the Lord, I am sorry; but I cannot stop loving Him and living for Him because He gave me back my life!" That was the last time I would go to that "Christian" counselor. It didn't take long for our marriage to take the downward spiral, and it eventually ended in 1996.

Children Wounded By Divorce

In the two years my marriage suffered through the pain of divorce and the ten years of battle since, I believe my children are the ones who have been wounded most. Children need stability and security. They want and desire for their parents to love each other. When there is fighting between two parents, whether that fighting is physical, verbal, mental or emotional, the children are definitely affected.

Children feel out of control because they can't stop the arguing and abuse. They are not allowed to talk and express their feelings because their feelings don't count. All that is important is what their parents want. It doesn't matter to the child who's right or who's wrong, all they know is that they want the arguing to stop.

How many times are children put in the middle of the battle, used like pawns in a chess game to see who will win? While working at Starbucks, I was witness to such an encounter. A couple was "discussing" who broke the visitation rules. As their daughter, who appeared to be around ten, sat at another table so she would not hear what was being discussed, the argument got pretty heated, and most everyone at Starbucks was aware of what was happening. The daughter went to her parents to try to calm the situation, but to no avail. Who really suffers the most through a scenario like this, if not the child?

What parents don't realize is the effect their divorce will have in how their children will view the world for the rest of their lives. Their faith and confidence in ever having their own good marriage is shattered, it affects their trust level and view of marriage, and eventually having children of their own. My twenty-six year old daughter, Christina, told me that having a happy marriage is a fantasy after living through the pain of our divorce. How very sad.

Christina wrote a poem that expressed her feelings at age fourteen. I cried when I read this poem because it was so revealing and had so much depth of emotion for someone so young. This poem was published in the 1997 edition of Keepsakes.

Eyes

Understanding, loving eyes, clearly shining
Over hurting friends, frail like decrepit flowers hanging
Their petals down toward the earth and yearning for
Some sunlight to give salvation and support

Deep wounded eyes, suffering miserably
For the events witnessed in past times; times when it would suffice
To say that these eyes were small innocent children who unbelievably
Have seen so much; they are weary and endeavor to see no more

Confused seeking eyes like one who sometimes tries to offer
Help if possible, but may pause or be precarious
Because of what is in front of him
Grateful eyes are as shining silver coins in the sun's brightness
Eyes are the ones who affect the situation and make the difference

Is there a way to influence others and
Give them help by the way of my eyes, or
Will I be blind?

When my youngest daughter, Stephanie, was a senior, she wrote a paper for her Composition class. The paper clearly shows who suffers the most by divorce.

What Happened To Christmas?

Eggnog, fireplaces, sledding, and snowsuits ought to be my Christmastime memories, but sadly enough, childhood dreams of waking up to presents and breakfast haven't always been part of my past. The Christmas I used to know has been blotted out, and replaced by complicated, distressful, and difficult Christmas seasons. While most families are recounting the wonderful Christmases of the past, my family makes an effort to look ahead, hoping this Christmas will bring more joy than tears.

As a child, I was blessed to have picture-perfect Christmases. My father, mother, sister and I would all spend a Saturday afternoon dressing up the fake Christmas tree with our favorite ornaments while listening to traditional Christmas music. My sister and I would take turns singing along with our favorite carols at the top of our lungs until it was time to put the angel on top of the tree. Although we alternated years, regarding whose turn it was, one of us would end up crying, jealous of the other who was granted this special privilege. We spent Christmas Eve in front of the fire, reading the story of Jesus' birth and, once again, singing at the top of our lungs to our favorite Christmas carols--except this time it was usually accappella.

However, all of that changed when I was 9 years old and my parents were divorced. Suddenly, Christmas became more difficult than ever. Setting up the Christmas tree wasn't the same without my dad there to stand it up straight. It didn't seem as special to put the angel on top of the tree anymore, especially since we were too big for my mom to lift us up high enough to reach the top anyway. It was heartbreaking to spend the holidays as a broken family.

One Christmas morning we had opened the presents with my mom and suddenly my dad was banging on the door, yelling for me to let him in. Apparently he thought it was time for us to go with him for Christmas. All I remember is standing in the dining room hearing my mom sobbing in the kitchen, begging me not to answer the door, while my dad was crying outside for me to let him in because he loved me and wanted to see me. I watched him walk away from the door and back to his car.

Christmas time since then hasn't been any easier. While my sister and I are with my dad and step mom, we put on a smile and pretend as if we've grown up in a perfect family. We don't bring up the past or the hard times. While we're with my mom, we'll still play the traditional Christmas music while setting up the tree, but it always reminds us of the pain. The hard times seem to come back to haunt us.

The past few Christmases have seemed to be as much of a struggle as those years ago. On Christmas Eve of my sophomore year, my mom received a call that she had breast cancer. Christmas of my junior year was spent driving to Florida with shingles up my side. This past Christmas we moved my sister to Kentucky and found out my mom had cancer once again. None of these events resulted in joyous laughter or happy memories.

Although the majority of the Christmases haven't been picture perfect for my family, we've managed to get through. The hard times have forced our family to completely rely on God for our strength. Christmas will never be as it once was to me, but Christ will always be the same. Through the tears and heartache, I still have a family; it may be a broken family, but it's a family nonetheless--and for that, I'm grateful.

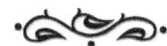

Life After Divorce

Is there hope for life after divorce? I say unequivocally, yes! God is able to take all of the bad and turn it around for our good. God is the only one that can heal our wounds, restore our trust, give us back our joy, and give us confidence for a new beginning.

Romans 8:28 NKJV - And we know that all things work together for good to those who love God, to those who are the called according to His purpose.

Psalms 34:18 – 19 - The Lord is close to the brokenhearted and saves those who are crushed in spirit. A righteous man may have many troubles but the Lord delivers him from them ALL.

Psalms 147:3 - He heals the brokenhearted and binds up their wounds.

Psalms 55: 22 - Cast your cares on the Lord and He will sustain you: He will never let the righteous fall.

Jeremiah 29:11 -"For I know the plans I have for you," declares the Lord. "Plans to prosper you and not to harm you; plans to give you hope and a future."

Isaiah 41: 10 – 13 - So do not fear, for I am with you; do not be dismayed, for I am your God. I will strengthen you and help you; I will uphold you with my righteous right hand. For I am the LORD, your God, who takes hold of your right hand and says to you, do not fear; I will help you.

Isaiah 26:3 NLT - You will keep in perfect peace all who trust in you, all whose thoughts are fixed on you!

Isaiah 51:12 - I, even I, am He who comforts you.

Matthew 11:28 – 30 - Come unto me, all you who are weary and burdened and I will give you rest. Take my yoke upon you and learn from me, for I am gentle and humble in heart and you will find rest for your souls. For my yoke is easy and my burden is light.

The scripture that I continue to claim for restoration is:

Joel 2:25 - I will restore to you the years that the locust have eaten.

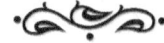

A New Beginning

I found myself crushed, bruised, and devastated; a single mother of two beautiful daughters living in a small community that clearly was "his town." If I stayed, I knew I would continue to spiral into an abyss from which I would not be able to escape. But God opened doors for us to move to a larger city. I had two typewritten pages of Scripture and confirmation that we were to move, but the final determination was that God had answered both of my daughters' fleeces about the move. The last fleece was when Stephanie said she would "know it is God if our home sells in a month." That would be proof that God wanted us to move. Well, God sold the house in three weeks. That was definite confirmation that we were to go forward.

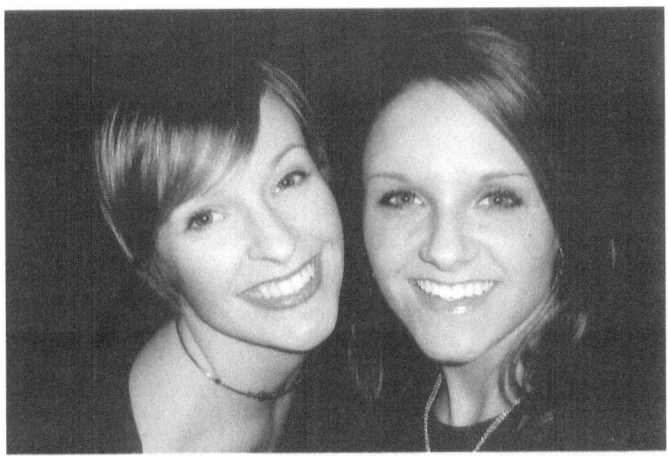

My beautiful daughters, Christina (left) and Stephanie (right)

What is a "fleece?" It comes from the story found in _Judges 6_. Gideon felt unqualified and thought God must have made a mistake, so he asked God for proof that he was to be the leader. Then God told Gideon to head up the fight against the Midianites.

Judges 6:36-40 - _Gideon said to God, "If you will save Israel by my hand as you have promised - look, I will place a wool fleece on the threshing floor. If there is dew only on the fleece and all the ground is dry, then I will know that you will save Israel by my hand, as you said." And that is what happened. Gideon rose early the next day; he squeezed the fleece and wrung out the dew—a bowlful of water._

Then Gideon said to God, "Do not be angry with me. Let me make just one more request. Allow me one more test with the fleece. This time make the fleece dry and the ground covered with dew." That night God did so. Only the fleece was dry; all the ground was covered with dew.

Friends told me they couldn't believe I would move my entire life, daughters, and business to a city where I knew no one. My response was, "What would be scary is to _not_ move when I have been clearly given so many signs that I must move. That would be total disobedience to His leading."

Proverbs 3:5 - _Trust in the Lord with all your heart and lean not on your own understanding. In all your way acknowledge Him and He will make your path straight._

Philippians 4:13 - _I can do all things through Christ who strengthens me._

Philippians 4:19 NKJV - _And my God shall supply all my needs according to His riches in glory by Christ Jesus._

Luke 8:31 - _Seek ye first the kingdom of God and His righteousness; and all these things shall be added unto you._

The move was the beginning of healing for my daughters and myself. God was 'lookin' out for our best interest and He knew what direction we needed to go. He provided us with a beautiful home and many new friends. We needed to be sensitive to His leading and follow in faith that there was a better plan.

We started attending an awesome church that helped in the healing process. I became the leader of the singles ministry and both of my daughters transitioned well into a school system that was four times larger than they were used to. Christina was in the marching band and on the dance team for three years. Stephanie played volleyball and was also on the dance team. What I loved most was the spiritual growth all three of us experienced. They say home is where the heart is and this new place quickly became our "home."

I had stopped singing during those years because I needed to heal. I kept saying the ministry was over because a lot of churches will not allow you to serve as a divorced woman, but God opened doors for me to share my testimony twice in 2001. I was so excited to think that perhaps the ministry was not over, only to find that I now had breast cancer. I would stop singing again until 2005 because I was presented another devastating blow.

Chapter Five

Breast Cancer

Cancer!

Amazing how this one small word can grip your heart with paralyzing fear. Until I heard that word, divorce was the most devastating thing I had experienced. But God's peace that passes all understanding would sustain me through both.

My journey began at 7:30 p.m. on Friday before New Year's Eve, 2001. I received a call from the nurse telling me that I had breast cancer. I specify the date and time because I want you to realize I had a long four-day holiday weekend with no one to answer any of my questions. At first, I started to panic, and then I immediately began to feel a peace, starting at the top of my head and flowing down through my entire body. Once again, God gave me just what I needed when I needed it. His watchful eye saw my need for His peace that passes understanding (*Philippians 4:7*). If God had not intervened supernaturally, I know I would have lost it.

I chose to have a lumpectomy with radiation in January 2002 because the tumor was small and close to the skin. When I arrived at the hospital, I believed they would not have to perform the surgery because everyone was joining me in prayer for God's healing. I was stunned to find that the tumor was still there and that we would proceed with the surgery. Everything went well and the report was great!   It was a stage one tumor with no node involvement, the best prognosis a woman can get when faced with breast cancer. Why then, did I have to endure seven surgeries in six years?

When I went for the radiation, I was told I had no insurance coverage for the $26,000 procedure. I could not believe this was happening.   I had just switched insurance agencies, and I had told my new agent I needed the best coverage possible because I'd had three previous pre-cancer tumors removed from my fibrous right breast a few years earlier.

I called the insurance company and was told the agent no longer worked there. The insurance company asked what they could do to help because the rider for chemotherapy and radiation had not been added to the policy.

I decided to have a mastectomy with back reconstruction, which they would cover. After much thought and prayer, I also asked for removal of my right breast, because I sensed in my heart it was not free of cancer. The bi-lateral mastectomy surgery took eleven-and-a-half hours but I was out of the hospital in two days.

I did amazingly well in spite of being totally filleted, front and back. I found that I was allergic to the narcotics given to help with the pain and ended up using Motrin 3. Amazing how God allowed this non-narcotic drug to help ease the pain after such a horrendous surgery.

I never knew what a normal breast should feel like until after my bi-lateral mastectomy because my breasts had been filled with fibrocystic disease -- lumps that kept moving. I remember the first time I inspected the teaching-model breast with a simulated mass. The nurse said my breast should not feel like the lump. I laughed and said my breast had never felt that smooth. My entire breast felt like the lump. Since the bi-lateral mastectomy, the silicone implants feel exactly like the teaching model, very smooth with no lumps.

While I was in the hospital, I noticed gauze on my right breast. I questioned the doctor and was told they had debated for over an hour about whether to sew the nipple back on because they had seen a suspicious spot. Why would there be a debate of putting the nipple back on if they saw something suspicious? I informed him the nipple area was where one of my three pre-cancerous tumors had been located. We were not sure if the tissue would live, so I kept saying, "Die you sucker, die," but the tissue did live. When the pathology report came back, it showed my right breast was full of carcinoma in situ, which is cancer that has not yet spread. My third surgery in four months would be to remove the nipple the doctors had chosen to put back on.

Second Tumor And Complications

The year 2002 continued to be very hard for me – my oldest daughter had a root canal and my youngest daughter had foot surgery. All three of us had accidents during one three-month period, and none of them were our fault. It was a funny sight when I opened the garage door to see my daughters' cars sitting there side-by-side with the passenger door dented on one and the driver's door dented on the other. Sometimes only a sense of humor can get you through the day!

That year dealt more blows as my dishwasher, washer and dryer, upright freezer, the sump pump and it's backup battery went out...all died on me. A water pipe burst because I left the lawn hose attached to the outside faucet during the winter. The largest expense was a new roof. I should have been a basket case; but still, I had God's peace that passes all understanding to see me through. The financial burden alone should have done me in, but God would "provide all of my needs according to His riches in glory" (*Philippians 4:19*). I felt as though God was carrying me just like in the poem, "Footprints."

Just when I thought things could not get any worse, I was hit with more devastating news, which made 2003 more challenging than 2002. Within a two-and-a-half month period, my father passed away, I moved Christina to Louisville for a job as a professional ballroom dance instructor, my brother John passed away, and then found that I had breast cancer once again. That year, I didn't have the peace God had given me in 2002.

I had shown two surgeons a lump at my three- and six-month checkups but was told not to worry because it was "scar tissue from my drains." I told them the drains had been under my arms, but was once again reassured not to worry. Big mistake. This "scar tissue" ended up being the original tumor, which had been left in my body because the doctors didn't remove the original biopsy trail site. (The original biopsy trail site is when they initially snip a piece of the "suspicious" area to find out if it is cancer.) This second tumor was now two-and-a-half times the size of my original tumor.

The one-month wait to coordinate the doctors' schedules was pure hell for me. Fear gripped my heart because my future was unsure. I didn't have God's peace as I had in 2002. A friend shared with me an acronym for the word *fear*: F.E.A.R. – False Evidence Appearing Real. I love this acronym because it is so very true. It helped to calm my fear, but I still had a lot of questions.

I don't understand why tissue at a biopsy trail site would ever be left in the body after all of the breast tissue has been removed. In fact, after finding out the doctors had not removed the trail site tissue, I contacted five breast cancer clinics across the country to ask their procedure in handling a biopsy trail site. Each clinic said that the biopsy trail site is always removed, especially when a mastectomy is involved. The doctors kept trying to tell me it was a recurrence. I always responded that it was *not* a recurrence, but it was the same tumor they left in my body.

Why did I go to the extreme of having both breasts removed, when the surgeon's policy of not removing the trail-site tissue, because "it is so rare for cancer cells to be dropped," would endanger my life? Would I live or die? Would their decision to leave in the trail-site tissue cut my life expectancy? Why would God allow this to happen? I later realized how God would use this "mistake" to heal the deepest wound to my soul…. the pain of my divorce.

God was faithful, for the tumor was encapsulated in scar tissue, thus keeping it from spreading. Even though the cancer had not spread, because the tumor had been left in, my chances for recurrence had risen to 38%. I had no choice but to have radiation since that procedure would bring the chance for recurrence down to 8%. This was still a $26,000 expense and the cost was still mine to pay.

The radiation caused my body to see the implant as a foreign object, so my body did what it was designed to do. It formed a capsule around the implant in an effort to kill the foreign object. In doing so, the implant got smaller and smaller and harder and harder. I affectionately called it "the incredible shrinking boob."

The implant had to be removed. My fifth surgery, a tram flap, (transverse rectus abdominis muscle), was done on March 14, 2007. This was by far the worst surgery of the five. They cut me from hipbone to hipbone, took muscle and fat from my stomach, put it under my skin and placed it where the breast mound is located. My stomach, in essence, is now my breast. It's like taking your lip and pulling it up over your head. Having experienced both types of reconstruction, I would highly suggest the back reconstruction with implants because the recovery and therapy time is minimal, not to mention the pain is much less with the back as compared to the abdominal pain.

When going through hard times that we don't understand, it may not be a time for God to show us how faithful He is to us, but rather to see how faithful we are to Him. Do we get angry and blame God or run into His arms like a hurting child knowing and trusting that "Daddy God" can make it better? My choice will always be to trust God because the world has nothing to offer. The worst time with the Lord is better than the best time in the world.

A Friend's Comfort And Concern

While I struggled to make sense of why I had a second tumor, a dear friend sent me a story that God used to help me process the questions I had about why I was going through this storm a second time. This is the email in its entirety.

THE ANT AND THE CONTACT LENS
A true story by Josh and Karen Zarandona
(Reprinted from Elisabeth Elliot newsletter, used by permission Elisabeth Elliot.org)

Brenda was a young woman who was invited to go rock climbing. Although she was very scared, she went with her group to a tremendous granite cliff. In spite of her fear, she put on the gear, took hold of the rope, and started up the face of that rock.

She got to a ledge where she could take a breather. As she was hanging on there, the safety rope snapped against Brenda's eye and knocked out her contact lens. Well, here she is, on a rock ledge, with hundreds of feet below her and hundreds of feet above her. Of course, she looked and looked and looked, hoping it had landed on the ledge, but it just wasn't there. Here she was, far from home, her sight now blurry. She was desperate and began to get upset, so she prayed to the Lord to help her to find it.

When she got to the top, a friend examined her eye and her clothing for the lens, but there was no contact lens to be found. She sat down, despondent, with the rest of the party, waiting for the rest of them to make it up the face of the cliff.

She looked out across range after range of mountains, thinking of that verse that says, "The eyes of the Lord run to and fro throughout the whole earth." She thought, "Lord, You can see all these mountains. You know every stone and leaf, and You know exactly where my contact lens is. Please help me."

Finally, they walked down the trail to the bottom. At the bottom there was a new party of climbers just starting up the face of the cliff. One of them shouted out, "Hey, you guys! Anybody lose a contact lens?" Well, that would be startling enough, but you know why the climber saw it? An ant was moving slowly across the face of the rock, carrying it on it's back.

Brenda told me that her father is a cartoonist. When she told him the incredible story of the ant, the prayer, and the contact lens, he drew a picture of an ant lugging that contact lens with the words, "Lord, I don't know why You want me to carry this thing. I can't eat it, and it's awfully heavy. But if this is what You want me to do, I'll carry it for You."

I think it would probably do some of us good to occasionally say, "God, I don't know why you want me to carry this load. I can see no good in it and it's awfully heavy. But, if you want me to carry it, I will."

God doesn't call the qualified, He qualifies the called. Yes, I do love GOD. He is my source of existence and my Savior. He keeps me functioning each and every day. Without Him, I am nothing, but with Him . . . I can do all things through Christ which strengthens me. (*Phil. 4:13*)

(Brenda I ~ Missed you in SAM class last Sunday. Someone emailed me this story. I thought about it quite a bit. God wanted the ant to carry something so that someone else could see it more clearly and find it. I do not know if this means anything to you, but I just felt led to send it to you. I am praying for you that God gives you strength, understanding and that He gives you answers to the questions that you have. I am wanting and praying for a physical healing for you. ~ Susan)

P.S. The use of the name "Brenda" in the above story is a coincidence. That is how it was emailed to me.

Since going through the breast cancer, my mortality has come to the forefront in my life. I have let go of the pain from my divorce and press on with gusto as I face each new day. Most of the time, my extreme Type A personality takes over and I get involved with far too many projects. I am passionate about life and passionate about living each day that God grants me to it's fullest. I don't know when I will take my last breath, but I will definitely make the most of this moment in time that I have been given.

I am thrilled to say the latest results of my PET scan, CT scan, and blood work prove that I am cancer FREE. I don't know what my future holds, but I certainly do know who holds my future. I know He will continue to walk with me through any storm I face. I trust Him because He is faithful!

Carrots, Eggs, And Coffee

Author Unknown

A young woman told her mother how hard things had been for her, how she wanted to give up, and was tired of fighting and struggling. When one problem was solved, a new one arose. Her mother took her to the kitchen, filled three pots with water, and placed each on a high fire until they began to boil. In the first pot she placed carrots, in the second she placed eggs, and in the last she placed ground coffee beans. She let them sit and boil without saying a word.

In twenty minutes she turned off the burners, fished the carrots out and placed them in a bowl. She pulled the eggs out and placed them in a bowl. Then she poured the coffee into a bowl. She asked her daughter, "Tell me what you see." "Carrots, eggs, and coffee," she replied.

Her mother asked her to feel the carrots. She did and noted that they were soft. The mother then asked the daughter to break the egg. She observed the egg was hardboiled. Finally, the mother asked the daughter to sip the coffee. The daughter smiled as she tasted its rich aroma. The daughter then asked, "What does it mean, mom?"

Her mother explained that each of these objects had faced the same adversity: boiling water. Each reacted differently. 1) The carrot went in strong, hard, and unrelenting. However, after being subjected to the boiling water, it softened and became weak. 2) The egg had been fragile. Its thin outer shell had protected its liquid interior, but after sitting through the boiling water, its inside became hardened. 3) The ground coffee beans were unique, however. After they were in the boiling water, they had changed the water.

"Which are you?" she asked her daughter. "When adversity knocks on your door, how do you respond? Are you a carrot, an egg or a coffee bean?" Which am I? Am I the carrot that seems strong, but with pain and adversity do I wilt and become soft and lose my strength? Am I the egg that starts with a pliable heart, but changes with the heat? Did I have a fluid spirit, but after a death, a breakup, a financial hardship or some other trial, have I become hardened and stiff? Does my shell look the same, but on the inside am I bitter and tough with a stiff spirit and a hardened heart? Or am I like the coffee bean? The bean actually changes the hot water, the very circumstance that brings the pain. When the water gets hot, it releases the fragrance and flavor. If you are like the bean, when things are at their worst, you get better and change the situation around you. When the hour is the darkest and trials are their greatest do you allow God to take you to another level?"

May you have enough happiness to make you sweet, enough trials to make you strong, enough sorrow to keep you human and enough hope to make you happy. The happiest of people don't necessarily have the best of everything; they just make the most of everything that comes their way. The brightest future will always be based on a forgotten past; you can't go forward in life until you let go of your past failures and heartaches. Most importantly, know that you cannot change people, but you can change the way you handle adversity...which just might encourage others to strive for change.

When you were born, you were crying and everyone around you was smiling. Live your life so at the end, you're the one who is smiling and everyone around you is crying.

May we all be COFFEE!!!

Chapter Six

God's Grace Through Loss

I have learned to not take the people in my life for granted. Relationships are the most important aspect of my life. Money, possessions, and position in life cannot fulfill me the way relationships fulfill me. The most crucial relationship I have is with my heavenly Father. I know He can take the bad things in my life and turn them around for good. I'm secure in knowing and trusting that there is a purpose for everything that happens. We all need HOPE for our future and the assurance that God is the provider for everything we need.

Romans 8:28 – *And we know that all things work together for good to those who love God, to those who are called according to His purpose.*

Jeremiah 29:11 – *"For I know the plans I have for you," declares the Lord, "plans to prosper you and not to harm you, plans to give you hope and a future."*

Ecclesiastes 5:19-20 – *When God gives any man wealth and possessions and enables him to enjoy them, to accept his lot and be happy in his work - this is a gift of God. God keeps him occupied with gladness of heart.*

When I was at my lowest point after the divorce, I remember asking God, "What hope and what future?" He spoke gently to my spirit in that still, small voice and said, "Brenda, I am your hope and I am your future."

It's so easy to look at life in a fleshly way, since we live in the world, but God was reminding me that I must look to the spiritual realm and the plan He has set before me.

God gave me an acronym for *hope*: H.O.P.E - Healer Of Pain's Entanglement. I have no hope when I am entangled in the pain, whether that pain is emotional, physical or spiritual. *Man's way leads to a hopeless end...God's way leads to an endless hope.* Jesus is the only one who can heal the deep wounds of my soul and give me HOPE.

The greatest healing I have experienced throughout this five-year ordeal was when I learned to let go of the hurt and pain from my past. Studies show there is a direct link between disease and holding on to the pain and nursing your wounds. I have heard it said; *He who angers you, controls you.* Forgiveness is a very crucial and freeing part of getting disease out of my life. I wish forgiveness was a one-time event, but as Jesus told Peter in *Matthew 18:21-22* - *Then Peter came to Jesus and asked, "Lord, how many times shall I forgive my brother when he sins against me? Up to seven times?" Jesus answered, "I tell you, not seven times, but seventy times seven."*

Forgiveness has been a process for me. Every time I forgave, something else would come up that needed forgiveness. The best advise I ever received was that we should forgive every time we even think about the person that offended us, then we are continually forgiving until we no longer think about the offense. Dr. Laura Schlessinger made a statement in a January 2006 television interview that I thought was profound. "You can't be on your mission if you're still on your history." When I learned to truly forgive, to let go, and to put my past behind me, then I began to live again.

ISAIAH 43:18-19 – Forget the former things; do NOT dwell on the past. See, I am doing a NEW thing! Now it springs up; do you not perceive it? I am making a way in the desert and streams in the wasteland.

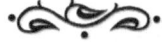

My Father's Passing

My father had a quadruple bi-pass with a pig mitral valve replacement at The Cleveland Clinic in 1987. I went to the Cleveland Clinic for four days to be with him and my mother during this time. I wanted to show him my love and concern. We talked for a long time the night before surgery and I was told he would "make things right with the Lord" if he made it through the surgery. God was faithful to bring my father through in great health, but he told me years later that he had not followed through with his promise.

We were told pig mitral valves last around twelve years before needing to be replaced. My father made it to sixteen years, to 2003, when his heart started to fail. He was in the hospital for five weeks before he passed away. We didn't learn that his heart was operating at ten percent capacity until after his death. God would use those five weeks to prepare my father for eternity.

I loved my father dearly, but he was very prejudiced, full of pride, had anger issues, and loved to argue over the Bible. While in the hospital, we saw my father's heart soften. His anger and pride disappeared as he became pliable in God's hands. My father was very weak due to the lack of oxygen to his body and would go in and out of consciousness. The day before he passed, he sat up in bed, opened his eyes, raised his hands toward heaven and softly spoke, "It's so beautiful." He lay back down in his bed peacefully, and went home to be with the Lord the next day. With God's watchful eye, He knew when and how to reach my father with His love. How wonderful is God's grace to change a hardened and prideful heart into one full of His love! God gave us the assurance that my father was now peacefully at home.

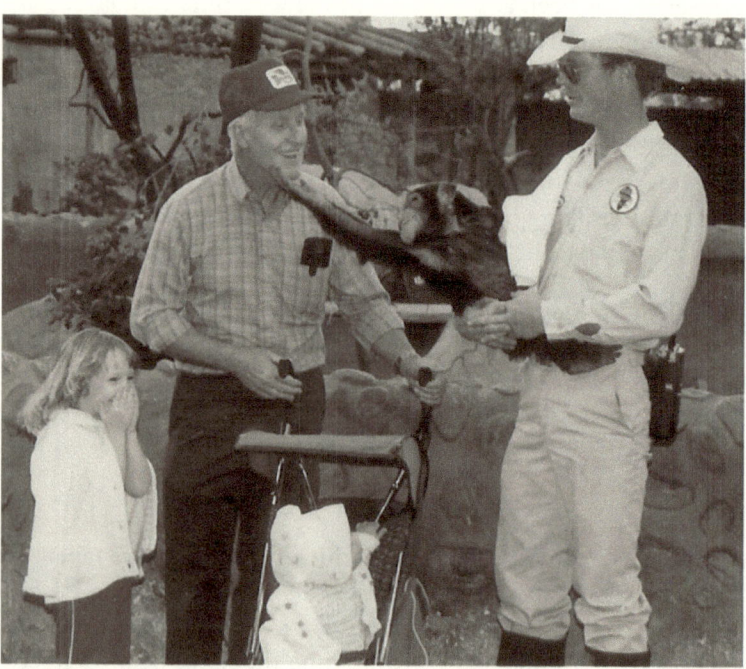

My favorite photo of dad at Busch Gardens with a monkey that adored him!

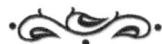

My Mother's Passing

God has taught me to value and savor each moment I am given to live life. He did this as I watched my mother in her battle with ovarian cancer in 2005. She was told she had three months to live, perhaps nine if she chose chemotherapy. She chose not to have chemo and lived a good quality of life for six of those nine months. She lived her last days with such peace, joy, dignity, and strength. People could not believe she was dying because she showed no signs for six months. She literally lived that scripture, *Psalms 23:4 – Yea, though I walk through the valley of the shadow of death, I will fear no evil for thou art with me; thy rod and thy staff they comfort me.* I watched as my mother walked through that valley.

When my mother found out the gravity of her situation, she told me not to pray for her healing because she wanted to go "home." I told her I would pray the same prayer for her as I pray for myself, "Lord, do not allow the enemy to take us out until the moment you have ordained for us to come home." I choose to live life just like my mother, with peace, joy, dignity, and strength. I do not know what the future may hold but I do know who holds my future!

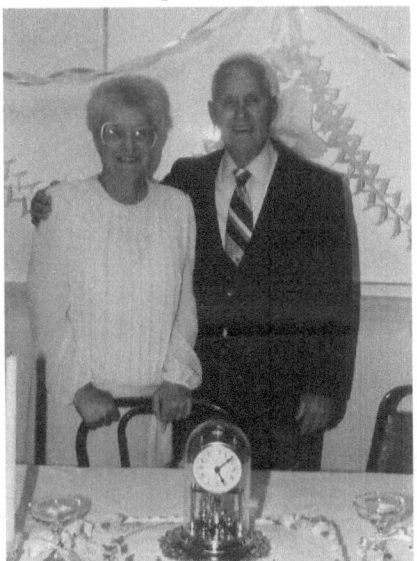

Mom & Dad's 50th Wedding Anniversary

I wake up each morning saying: "Good morning Lord," instead of "Good Lord, it's morning." Attitude is crucial to living a successful life. I don't want to just make a living…I want to make a life. I want my life to count for something just like my mother. I want to fulfill my purpose and hear Him say to me when I see Him face to face, as in *Matthew 25:21 - 'Well done, good and faithful servant! You have been faithful with a few things; I will put you in charge of many things. Come and share your master's happiness!'*

There is a saying I love: *Life is a gift…that's why it's called the Present!* The word present has two meanings – a gift God has given to me; and present – this present moment of time. Today is all we have. We are not guaranteed tomorrow. We need to make the most of God's gift now! I have a plaque that reads: God's *gift to you is who you are. Your gift to God is who you become.*

My favorite saying is: *"Life is not measured by the number of breaths we take, but by the moments that take our breath away."*

Dealing With Loss

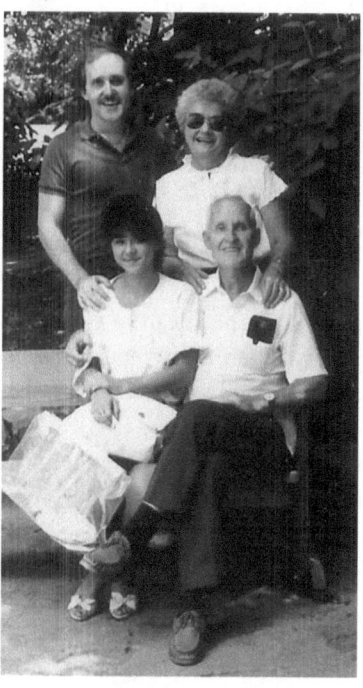

John, Julia (John's daughter), Mom & Dad

With all that had happened in a short five-year period, I felt a lot like Job. I would quote *Job 13:15 KJV* - *Though He slay me, yet will I trust in Him.* Every time I needed to be encouraged, God was faithful to speak to me through His Word, have someone call and speak words of "life" into my spirit, or He would lead me to inspirational illustrations to show me He was still there. The will of God will never take you where the grace of God will not protect you.

Having friends and family is crucial to getting out of the pit of despair. I love the saying: *People don't care how much you know until they know how much you care.* True living comes when you are surrounded with people who love and care for you. That is what brings real healing.

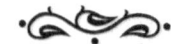

Powerful Squash

At Amherst College, researchers experimented with a squash seed that had been planted in rich, fertile soil. Eventually, the seed produced a squash as big as a soccer ball. Then the researchers placed a steel band around the squash. Attached to the steel band was a device for measuring "lifting power." The purpose of the experiment was to determine the lifting power of the squash. As the squash continued to grow and stretch the steel band, it reached a lifting power of 500 pounds. Amazing!! Within two months, the lifting power went up to 1,500 pounds. A month later it was 2,000 pounds.

It was not until the lifting power had reached an incredible 5,000 pounds that the rinds broke.

When the squash was opened, the researchers discovered that it had built up a whole network of tough fibers to fight against the pressure that was binding its growth. Moreover, the roots supporting the squash had reached out over 80,000 feet in every direction searching for more and more nourishment to strengthen the fibers.

How do we handle tough times? What do we do when we are put under great pressure? I truly believe that it's during those times that God gives us "lifting power" to strengthen us, just like that squash. He uses those tough times to make our roots go deeper into His grace and His ability to help us to withstand hard times. I believe the whole network of tough fibers used to fight against the pressure that was binding its growth is similar to our network of support from friends and family. *You can give without loving but you can't love without giving.* As they gave me their support, they proved their love for me.

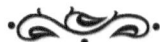

The Turn-Around

God brings people in and out of our lives for His special purpose. August 2005 was a turning point in my life and in my ministry. I was still struggling with low self-esteem, not knowing who I was, and what my purpose was for living. My promotional products business was going well and I had started a part-time job at Starbucks for benefits. Working at Starbucks opened up many opportunities for me to meet awesome people who God would use in my life. I met a beautiful woman who was a kindred spirit. In our conversation, as she ordered her latte, I found that her husband was a pastor and that God had blessed her financially through owning McDonald franchises. When she found out I was a singer, she invited me to share at her husband's Pastor Appreciation Night.

This night was presented as "Oscar Night." It was held at the Embassy Theater in Fort Wayne, catered by Catablu, a wonderful American cuisine restaurant. It was a black tie affair, with everything done first class. As I introduced myself to those at my table, I noticed that everyone had their doctorate degree. I started to feel myself slump into my chair, feeling "less than" because I was just Brenda, not Dr. Brenda.

The two gentlemen who emceed the evening had worked with many secular stars, such as Usher.   Again, I felt myself slump deeper, feeling smaller still.   Why was I here?   I didn't feel that I belonged.   Then a women's group sang that was phenomenal.   I kept feeling smaller and smaller inside, wondering what God could possibly be thinking by having me sing for this event.   The enemy has a way of making us feel "less than" especially when comparing ourselves to those around us.   Even though I know we are told not to compare, I couldn't help but feel insignificant, and that I had nothing to offer.   _Galatians 6:4 – Each one should test his own actions. Then he can take pride in himself without comparing himself to someone else._

I went to the restroom to freshen my lipstick before I sang.   I prayed as I talked to God about what was going on, like He didn't know.   I told Him that even though I didn't feel as if I belonged, I knew He had opened the door and I asked Him to show me why I was there.   I sang, "All In Favor" by Larnelle Harris and the response was overwhelming!

When I got back to the table there was a woman who had come in late so I introduced myself to her.   She remarked that my song was "off the chain."   I thanked her, and then told her I wished everyone could know what a miracle it was that I could even sing.   I shared the rest of my testimony with her and she said I could have given my testimony in thirty seconds: "I had throat surgery and was told I would never sing again, I went through a devastating divorce that wiped out my ministry for eight years, and satan tried to take me out two times through breast cancer, but God had a plan.   God always has a plan.   All of those in Favor, say 'I'."   I was blown away at how God used Rhonda in my life that night and for the next two years.

At the end of the program, the pastor began ministering with such an anointing that people were being "slain" in the spirit.   I like to describe this experience as having God's spirit come over you so gently that you cannot stand before His presence.   You are aware of everything going on around you, but your body is "still" before the Lord.   It's as though you are in God's operating room and He is performing spiritual surgery on you.   He is removing thoughts, attitudes, and things that do not belong while replacing them with what is necessary to help you live the life He has planned.   This happened to my niece, Julia, when she was just six years old.   She lay "still" for almost an hour.   Only God could keep a six-year-old "still" for that amount of time.

I was standing alone watching God move through this man.   He was about 20 feet from me when he stopped, opened his eyes, looked at me, closed his eyes again and pointed his finger toward me.   He gave me this message, "I know the hurt and pain you have had in your life. I know the rejection you have faced. I know the many times you have said it was over. You keep saying it is over and you believe it is over, but God is here to tell you, "It's not over till God says it's over." He will use you to bring healing into those He brings into your life." I sat down and cried because it wasn't this man speaking to me, but it was God speaking. I had never told anyone that I felt the ministry was over; only God knew what I had said.

I knew this was a message directly from the throne of God to me and it was my turn-around for the ministry. You see, the enemy wants to get us down and keep us down anyway he can. Satan knows our weaknesses and will use those weak areas against us, but God desires to build us up in the midst of our pain and misery. God is the only one that gives us a new beginning. He gives us a future and is our hope! *Jeremiah 29:11* As I said earlier, He is our HOPE – Healer Of Pain's Entanglement. God is always 'lookin' over His children with love and protection.

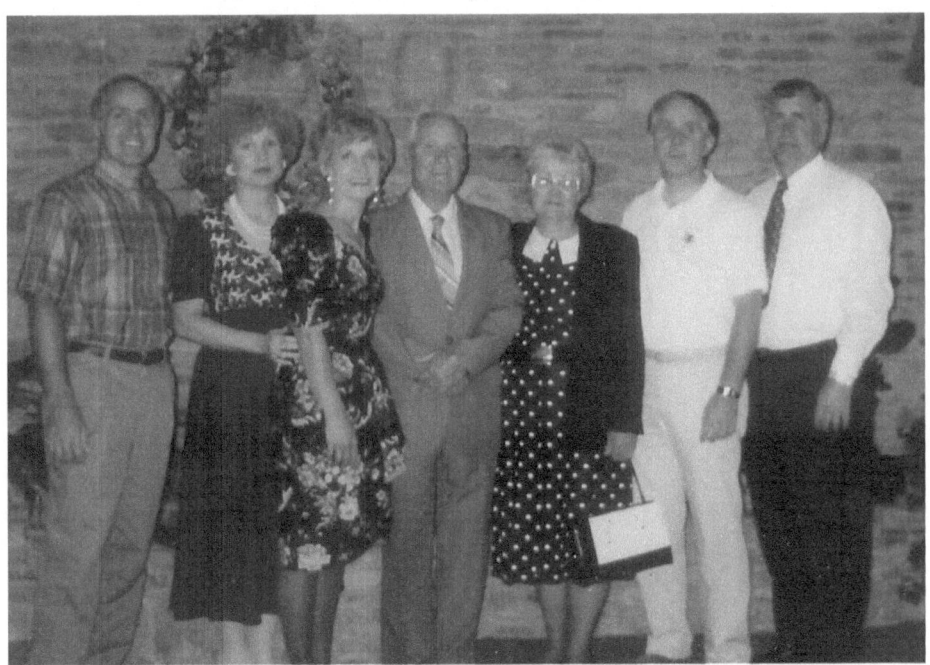

Our last family photo taken in 1995. I absolutely LOVE the hair and puff sleeves ☺☺
Left to right: Gregg, Pam, Me, Dad, Mom, John and Jim

I prayed God would give me original material for my new CD project, "Refined Hope." He gave me the words to "It's Not Over Till God Says It's Over" based on that divine appointed evening.

It's Not Over Till God Says It's Over

April 15, 2006

It's not over till God says it's over
It's not over cause God's got a plan
It's not over till God says it's over
Trust in the Lord as He holds your hand

Disappointments and discouragements too deep to bear
A lifetime of losses, so why should I dare
To trust and believe there's a plan for my good
When everything is shattered and misunderstood?

Crushed, I'm so crushed that's all I can feel
Oh, God speak to my heart and let me know you are real
I cry for your presence and thirst after your spirit
I can't go on living unless you help me bear it

The plan I thought you had for my life
Was taken away and is now nowhere in sight
For years I've been thinking my dream was over
How could you use me, downtrodden and older?

Then you spoke to that secret place in my soul
Through a man who did not know me at all
You said, "I know what you've been through
I was there in your midst, your pain will
Bring healing to those that I draw

Your dream is not over for it came from me
From my heart to your heart, why can't you see?
My plan is much bigger than you'll every know
Just stand back in awe and watch it unfold

Now rest in my goodness, give me all of your cares
Trust me with your future for nothing compares
With the plans I have for good and not harm
I will lift you above with my almighty right arm

I tell you it's not over till I say it's over
It's not over cause I've got a plan
It's not over till I say it's over
For I am Alpha and Omega
The Beginning and the End!"

Chapter Seven

In the Midst of the Pain

I have learned during my lifetime that pain is relative. When I was a child and had all of the accidents, I experienced pain. When I developed hepatitis A during the summer before fourth grade, I hated to get shots each week because of the pain. I remember running around the table three or four times before they were able to catch me to administer the shot. I didn't want to feel that sharp pain again even though it was necessary to get better.

I have had people tell me how they would never complain again about what they were going through after finding out what I had experienced. My response is, NEVER compare your pain to anyone else's. Pain is pain and it hurts just the same whether it is physical, mental or emotional. The pain you are going through is just as hurtful as the pain I am going through, different, but still pain and still very hard to deal with.

The needles I endured as a child were nothing compared to the pain of the eleven-and-a-half hour bi-lateral mastectomy recovery; and that recovery was nothing compared to the eight-hour tram flap recovery I experienced in March 2007. However, neither of those recoveries was as painful as the emotional pain of the divorce and the emotional pain I felt after discovering the doctors had left the second tumor in my body.

Psalms 34:18-19 — *The Lord is close to the broken hearted and saves those crushed in spirit. A righteous man has many troubles but the Lord delivers him from them all.*

Psalms 147:3 — *He heals the brokenhearted and binds up their wounds.*

No matter what pain we are dealing with, what is crucial is how we work through the pain. Do we get angry with God and take our anger out on those around us? I must say, there were times I did just that. There were times I got angry with God and I told Him so. I'm so thankful that nothing I experience takes Him by surprise. He did not fall off His throne when I went through the divorce or when I found out about the cancer. He certainly did not wipe me off the face of the planet because I got mad at Him. He knows what we are thinking so we need to just be honest with Him and tell him every feeling we have. This allows Him to help us work through the pain, to not take our anger out on our loved ones, and to "carry" us, if necessary, as we process the pain.

1 Peter 5:7 NKJV - *Casting all your cares upon Him, for He cares for you.*

Philippians 4:6 -7 NKJV — *Be anxious for nothing, but in everything by prayer and supplication, with thanksgiving, let your request be made known to God; and the peace of God, which passes all understanding, will guard your hearts and minds through Christ Jesus.*

I have tried to live by the saying: *When you get to the end of your rope, tie a knot and hold on,* but there were times when the pain was so great that I could not hold on. If God had not been faithful in holding onto me, I know I wouldn't have made it. There were times when I could not even pray another word because of the despair and pain. It was during those times, I know, that people interceded with the Lord on my behalf through their prayers.

Any time God puts someone on your heart or brings them to your mind, please pray for them at that moment because you don't know what God may be doing. Prayer is key to setting into motion the angelic beings and the plan God desires to work in our lives.

James 5:16 NKJV — *The effectual fervent prayer of a righteous man avails much.*

Matthew 7:7 - *Ask and it will be given to you; seek and you will find; knock and the door will be opened to you.*

The encounter between the Archangel Gabriel and Daniel shows how prayer will start the process of working God's plan. It also shows the battle that takes place in the spiritual realm to finally get the answers to prayer.

Daniel 10:12-14 - Then he (Gabriel) continued, "Do not be afraid, Daniel. **Since the first day** *that you set your mind to gain understanding and to humble yourself before your God, your words were heard, and I have come in response to them.* **But the prince of the Persian kingdom resisted me twenty-one days.** *Then Michael, one of the chief princes, came to help me, because I was detained there with the king of Persia. Now I have come to explain to you what will happen to your people in the future, for the vision concerns a time yet to come."*

Angelic beings are an intricate part of God's design. They have always been used for our protection, guidance, and bringing about God's plan as He continues to watch over us. There are many accounts where angels have made themselves available to be seen just as in the story of the Archangel Gabriel and Daniel. This is just another reason to treat everyone with kindness and respect, for you may be dealing with an angel.

Hebrews 13:2 - Do not forget to entertain strangers, for by so doing, some people have entertained angels without knowing it.

Our Spoken Words

The saying: *Sticks and stones may break my bones, but words will never hurt me*, is a lie right from the pit of hell. In fact, some of the deepest wounds I bear are not from the scalpel that cut deeply into my body, but from the very hurtful and cutting words spoken to my soul. You never see these "wounds" but they are there and it may take years to even begin the healing process. My healing process did not start until I sought out good Christian counseling. It took four years to "peel back the layers" and get to the "root" of the pain so the healing could begin.

Proverbs 12:18 – Reckless words pierce like a sword, but the tongue of the wise brings healing.

Proverbs 15:1 – A gentle answer turns away wrath but a harsh word stirs up anger.

Proverbs 15:4 – The tongue that brings healing is a tree of life, but a deceitful tongue crushes the spirit.

Proverbs 18:21 – The tongue has the power of life and death.

Proverbs 4:24 – Put away perversity from your mouth, keep corrupt talk from your lips.

I try to live by *Ephesians 4:29 –30 – Do not let any unwholesome talk come out of your mouth, but only what is helpful for building others up according to their needs – do not grieve the Holy Spirit.* This Scripture shows that we can actually grieve God's Holy Spirit by speaking mean, hurtful and demeaning words--to anyone.

Genesis 8:21 – every inclination of his (mankind) heart is evil from childhood.

Luke 6:45 – The good man brings good things out of the good stored up in his heart, the evil man brings evil things out of the evil stored up in his heart. For out of the overflow of his heart, his mouth speaks. Which one are you? Only God can change a person's heart from evil to good through the working of His Holy Spirit. He is lovingly waiting for those who desire to change.

I know one reason I have experienced so much pain is so that I will be able to listen and comfort others as they struggle to understand what they are going through. I specify the word "listen" because people in pain need the freedom to express what they are feeling without being told they are wrong for feeling this way or being told how to "fix" the problem. Listening is the best way to show your love to someone in pain.

2 Corinthians 1: 4 – Praise the God of all comfort, who comforts us in all our troubles, so that we can comfort those in any trouble with the comfort we ourselves have received from God.

This Scripture shows that we are each called to comfort others with the same comfort we have received from God. In the song "Comfort the People" on my CD "Change," the words deal very clearly with our call to reach out to those that are hurting.

COMFORT THE PEOPLE

Look around; it is never far see who the wounded people are
They are close to you, there is so much good your love can do

Look around; let compassion rise for every broken heart that cries
Bring them close to you; wrap them in His love forever true

CHORUS
Comfort the people, meet them with love
God is the hand and we are the glove
Jesus is reaching, we reach with Him
Go to the people and comfort them, comfort them

Look around, it is never far between yourself and a broken heart
Feel the pain they feel, feel His love that loves enough to heal

Worst Surgery Yet

This last surgery for the tram flap was the absolute worst surgery I have ever had. I was in ICU for five days. The doctor told me I would need 24/7 care after being released from the hospital. I told him my family was in Louisville and that I was living alone because Stephanie had moved out to be closer to college. He said he would put me in a rehab facility for two weeks so I would get the care I needed. However, I was "doing so well" that he sent me home.

I came home with drains on both sides of my hips from the hipbone-to-hipbone incision and also a drain in my breast. These had to be monitored for the amount of liquid my body was producing. I had to sleep in a recliner for six weeks and could barely move. Stephanie came home for my first week and did the best that she could, but she really didn't know what to do for me. I didn't even know what to ask her to do.

My first night home, I got out of the recliner, which was very difficult to do on my own, and went to the restroom. On my way out, I was feeling very disoriented and knew that I was going to fall. I was on the landing and had two choices for the fall: I could fall to the right and end up falling down my stairs to the basement, or I could fall to the left and fall into my wall mirror. I chose the mirror, which turned out to be the correct choice. I thank God for His protection in keeping me from injury.

When Stephanie left, I was alone -- and I do mean alone. I received plenty of get-well cards but most friends stayed away because they thought I was in rehab or they didn't want to disturb me. Please, please disturb me. My church family didn't contact me because my pastor had had surgery soon after mine; and the secretary who lets everyone know what's going on was out of commission also. There is nothing worse than being in physical pain, being unable to move, and feeling totally alone. The emotional despair was as bad, if not worse, than the physical pain. The enemy took full advantage of this and put me into a deep pit of depression.

At my lowest point, I managed to maneuver my body into my home office, sit in front of my computer, and "vent" all of my frustration, anger and disappointment at God. I banged away at the keyboard as I cried, questioning why I had to go through this again, what had I done to deserve this punishment, why was God mad at me, why had He abandoned me, and when would I ever "feel" His presence in my life again. Here is an excerpt of what I wrote that night.

I hate when people think I'm so strong, they have no clue what's hidden beneath my smile. The casual, "How are you doing today?" but do they really want to know the pain I'm feeling in the depth of my soul? Our lives are so fast-paced that no one has the time to sit and listen before they must leave for their next meeting.

Will this pain last just one day or will it linger on forever? What causes the pain to be worse one day than another? It's not just the physical pain I feel that's as bad as the pain of loneliness and knowing I am truly alone. Where do I go next at this last stage of my life, alone by myself with no one to help work through the choices I have?

I struggle between wanting to live and truly wanting to die. What purpose can I serve when I don't even know the answers to my questions about what I've been through? I know what your Word says about turning the bad things around for our good; but just when I felt I had gone to the next level, as people told me you were doing in my life, I'm hit with the biggest surgery of my life.

*I cry when I look at all of the scars on my body and wonder what man would possibly want to have me in his life? My left breast is so mutilated from the four surgeries. I'm told the scars will gradually disappear as time passes, **but will the scars in my soul do the same**?*

How many others feel this same way? After the physical scars fade, will the emotional scars to the soul fade away and eventually heal? I know that most of the emotional scars that have been carved into my life are from those closest to me. The enemy uses those "in our camp" to inflict wounds that we would never allow anyone else to inflict. People on the outside don't affect us, and are not given an in-road to our hearts the way our loved ones are. Therefore, who would be better for the enemy to use to make us feel as if we were unworthy, unloved, stupid, ignorant, and all of those other lies that are perpetrated upon us? For this one reason alone, we must know who we are in Christ. If we don't, we will be pulled down into a pit we might not be able to escape.

My value and worth are based solely upon Jesus Christ. Without Christ in my life, I am nothing. He wakes me up each morning, gives me life, and is my life-breath. He is my healer, He is my strength, He is my peace, He is my comfort, He is the one who gets me through the storm, and He guides my path as He directs my life. He gives me wisdom, provides my finances, is the Father to my children, and grants me favor with those I meet. I do not want God's permissive will in my life. I want His perfect will.

Jeremiah 10:23–I know, Oh Lord, that a man's life is not his own; it is not for man to direct his steps.

1 Chronicles 28:9 – Acknowledge the God of your father and serve Him with wholehearted devotion and with a willing mind, for the Lord searches every heart and understands every motive behind the thought. If you seek Him, He will be found by you; but if you forsake Him, He will reject you forever.

Romans 12:1-2 – Offer your bodies as living sacrifices, holy and pleasing to God – this is your spiritual act of worship. Do not conform any longer to the pattern of this world, but be transformed by the renewing of your mind. Then you will be able to test and approve what God's will is – His good, pleasing and perfect will.

After I "vented" my last frustration, I sat back in the chair and took a deep breath. I felt much better for having released my anger and disappointment. I sat looking at the computer then proceeded to write.

"Okay, so I don't "feel" your presence. It doesn't matter. I am not leaving you whether I feel your presence or not. I've been in the world and it has NOTHING to offer. You are the only one who can comfort me, give me peace in my life and fill me with joy. Even though I don't "feel" those things right now, I know I will. I know that one-day "this too shall pass." It's you and me. That's all I know!"

Sometimes the things we experience in life are to make us choose which path we will take. Happiness is a choice, looking at the glass as half full instead of half empty is a choice, putting on a smile instead of a frown is a choice, forgiveness is a choice, loving others is a choice. I have heard it said: *Hard times don't make or break you…they reveal the real you.* When things start to heat up, what's inside will come out.

While laying in the recliner, depressed and hurting physically and emotionally, I heard a song that so touched my heart. The song by Vicki Yohe titled, *In The Waiting*, was exactly what I needed to hear because it was what I was feeling at the time. I needed to know that I was not alone, that He knew where I was, and what I was experiencing. Her song addresses how God uses pain in our lives to make us stronger; but during the pain, we need to feel His peace that passes understanding, we need to know that He is in the middle of the our pain and hurting. Most of all, we need to rest in knowing it's okay to be 'in the waiting.'

God will use anything necessary to reach us with His love. First and foremost, He uses His written Word, the Bible, to let us know how much He loves us and cares about what is happening in our lives, but you must believe the Bible is God speaking directly to you.

In *Numbers 22:22-35* – God used a donkey to talk to Balaam, the prophet. This is quite an interesting read.

2 Timothy 3:16 - All Scripture is God-breathed and is useful for teaching, rebuking, correcting and training in righteousness.

Hebrews 4:12 – For the Word of God is living and active. Sharper than any double-edged sword, it penetrates even to dividing soul and spirit, joints and marrow; it judges the thoughts and attitudes of the heart.

Isaiah 55:11 - So is my word that goes out from my mouth: It will not return to me empty, but will accomplish what I desire and achieve the purpose for which I sent it.

Luke 21:33 – Heaven and earth will pass away, but my Words will never pass away.

Romans 10:17 NKJV – So then faith comes by hearing, and hearing by the Word of God.

Proverbs 4:20 –22 NLT – Listen carefully to my words. Don't lose sight of them. Let them penetrate deep into your heart, for they bring life to those who find them and healing to their whole body.

God uses music to minister to my soul. There are so many songs that uplift me in spite of my pain. I love to sing "Less Like Scars" written by Sarah Groves. Everything we go through is to conform us to the image of Jesus Christ so we take on more of His character.

LESS LIKE SCARS

It's been a hard year but I'm climbing out of the rubble
These lessons are hard, healing changes are subtle, but everyday it's
Less like tearing, more like building. Less like captive, more like willing
Less like breakdown, more like surrender. Less like haunted, more like
remember

CHORUS
And I feel You here and You're picking up the pieces,
You're forever faithful
Seemed out of my hands, a bad situation, but You are able
And in Your hands the pain and hurt look less like scars
and more like character

Less like a prison, more like my room.
It's less like a casket, more like a womb
Less like dying, more like transcending
Less like fear, less like an ending

Just a little while ago I couldn't feel the power or the hope,
I couldn't cope, I couldn't feel a thing
Just a little while back, I was desperate, broken, laid out,
hoping You would come

I don't know anyone who wants to struggle through pain or who wants to experience any horrendous circumstances that devastate them to the point of wanting to give up. However, I do know that pain serves a purpose in God's plan. There is a role that pain plays in our lives. Pain makes us aware that there is a problem. When we experience pain, it is important to forgive and put the pain behind us. However, it is also important to have a memory of the pain, so we will never allow ourselves to experience that pain again.

When a parent tells a child not to touch a hot stove, but the child touches the hot stove anyway, the pain the child feels will remain in his memory and keep him from touching the hot stove again. The same holds true with the pain of divorce. We can put the pain behind us, but we will definitely be determined to not make the same mistakes twice. Hopefully, we will enter marriage the second time wiser, more flexible, and more open to work on problems. Learning from past mistakes is crucial to our growth and becoming who God desires for us to be.

I love the saying: *God's gift to you is who you are. Your gift to God is who you become.* God loves me just as I am, but He loves me too much to leave me that way. I know with all my struggles through the years, I have grown. I know God has remained faithful, that He is always 'lookin' out for me, that He desires to heal me, that He cares for me, that He has a plan for me, and that He will keep me through the struggles for His good purpose. This "living life" thing is not about me at all; it's all about Him.

Philippians 1:6 NKJV – *Being confident of this very thing, that He who has began a good work in you will complete it until the day of Jesus Christ.*

Philippians 4:13 NKJV – *I can do all things through Christ who strengthens me.*

Philippians 4:19 NKJV – *And my God shall supply all my needs according to His riches in glory by Christ Jesus.*

Galatians 6:9 – *Let us not become weary in doing good, for at the proper time we will reap a harvest if we do not give up.*

Chapter Eight

John's Story

It amazes me that the same God who created the universe loves me so much and is concerned about every aspect of my life. He is all knowing and all seeing as His watchful, loving eyes keep 'lookin' out for us. God has worked in and through the circumstances of my life to show me He is always there whether I "feel" His presence or not. Even when people do not want Him in their life, He is there as long as someone is praying and interceding for that individual.

The most dynamic story of love, grace, mercy, forgiveness, and total deliverance I have ever heard is a true story in the life of my brother, John, who passed away in 2003 from a brain tumor. This story must be told because people need to know what a loving Father we have and the lengths He will go to in order to reach an unsaved soul.

Each of the children in my family had accepted Jesus Christ as our Savior at an early age but drifted away as we became teenagers. We could no longer use the cover of my mother's relationship to God to keep us in His good standing. The time comes when each of us must choose to remain in the faith even in the face of temptation to be drawn away. There is a defining moment when we will have to make a choice to stand strong or to cower down and fall, leaving God behind. When we no longer sense His presence, or His work in our lives, it is because we have moved away. He promises to never leave us nor forsake us (*Deuteronomy 31:6 and 8, Joshua 1:5*).

God's promise in *Proverbs 22:6 NKJV* – *Train a child in the way he should go, and when he is old, he will not depart from it* -- is exactly what happened to each of us. I was the first to return back to the Lord at the age of twenty-two. Within two-and-a-half years, my brothers, Gregg and Jim, along with my sister Pam returned also. The only one who stayed away was my brother, John. He was living a homosexual lifestyle.

We were each growing stronger in our faith with a steadfastness we had not experienced before, because as grownups we had chosen it. We were no longer going to church because our mother made us go. When we stand before Christ on judgment day, there will be no one standing with us, no excuses to be given, and everything will be revealed. Our thoughts, our motives, and our entire lives will be played before us as we stand before the one truly righteous Judge. Will we be found guilty of our sin or will our sins be covered and washed away by the blood that Jesus Christ shed on the cross?

Hebrews 9:27 KJV – *It is appointed unto men once to die, after this the judgment.*

Romans 14:10-12 NKJV – *For we shall all stand before the judgment seat of Christ. As surely as I live, says the Lord, every knee shall bow before me, and every tongue shall confess to God. So then each of us shall give account of himself to God.*

Matthew 12:36 – *But I tell you that men will have to give account on the day of judgment for every careless word they have spoken.*

Ecclesiastes 12:14 – *For God will bring every deed into judgment, including every hidden thing, whether it is good or evil.*

John was very musically gifted and talented. He was drum major and played the drums in the band during his high school days. While working in New Orleans, he was given the honor to conduct the New Orleans Orchestra. In Louisville, there was a contest to write a song about the steamboat, The Belle of Louisville. John composed, "The Ballad of the Belle," which was recorded and released as the winning song. It was very exciting for us to witness his success.

I'm not sure why John chose the homosexual lifestyle. Perhaps it was having an absentee father with a very dominant controlling mother or because older teenage boys molested him as a young child. I asked him one day about the statement that "he was born that way." He told me, "It is a lie from the pit of hell. I needed to believe the lie of being born that way or I would have to face the reality of my sin."

We tend to categorize sin, but the Word shows that we are all guilty of sin and that breaking even one of the Ten Commandments makes us guilty of breaking them all.

Romans 3:23 – For all have sinned and fall short of the glory of God.

James 2:10-11 - For whoever keeps the whole law and yet stumbles at just one point is guilty of breaking all of it. For he who said, "Do not commit adultery," also said, "Do not murder." If you do not commit adultery but do commit murder, you have become a lawbreaker.

The Good News is that Jesus Christ came to pay the price for our sin. He will stand beside us on Judgment Day and declare us "not guilty" if we have asked Him into our lives to be our Savior.

Romans 6:23 – For the wages of sin is death, but the gift of God is eternal life in Christ Jesus, our Lord.

Colossians 1:22 – But now He has reconciled you by Christ's physical body thru death to present you holy in His sight, without blemish and free from accusation.

Our sin is covered by the blood Jesus shed on the cross, to never be remembered any longer.

Isaiah 43:25 – I, even I, am He who blots out your transgression for my own sake and remembers your sins no more.

Hebrews 10:17 – Their sins and lawless acts I will remember no more.

Romans 8:1 – Therefore, there is now no condemnation for those who are in Christ Jesus, because through Christ Jesus the law of the Spirit of life set me free from the law of sin and death.

Psalm 103:12 – As far as the east is from the west, so far has He removed our transgressions from us.

John signed up to serve in the Air Force. While in Korea, he tried one last time to remain straight, having a relationship with a beautiful Korean girl named Yusuni. He married Sandy, her American name, and they had the most perfect baby I have ever seen, Julia. They were eagerly welcomed into our family. However, John could not resist the strong pull of homosexuality and was discharged from the Air Force.

John returned to Louisville with Sandy and Julia. They lived with my parents until they could find a place of their own. Sandy truly loved the person John was and prayed for him to be her faithful husband, but that was not to be. They divorced and John returned wholeheartedly into the homosexual community. For years we prayed for his turn-around. John wouldn't associate with our family because we were all Christians and all we talked about was the Lord and what He was doing in our lives. We never talked about John's homosexuality even though we all knew. We continued to love him and pray for him. We are called to "love the sinner, but hate the sin" as quoted by Mahatma Gandhi.

I remember the day I stopped praying for John. In my prayer time, I told the Lord that I was not going to pray for John any longer because he had chosen the homosexual lifestyle and I did not see how he could possibly change. My mother, however, would never give up believing in John's deliverance. She was just like the widow in Luke 18 who kept nagging until finally the judge gave her what she wanted. My mother prayed each of her children back into the Kingdom of God and she was not going to leave one behind.

Luke 18:2-5 - In a certain town there was a judge who neither feared God nor cared about men. And there was a widow in that town who kept coming to him with the plea, 'Grant me justice against my adversary.' For some time he refused, but finally he said to himself, 'Even though I don't fear God or care about men, yet because this widow keeps bothering me, I will see that she gets justice, so that she won't eventually wear me out with her coming!'

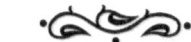

God's Deliverance

In 1985, my mother's prayers were answered. She called me to share how John had given her an ultimatum. He knew she had always loved him, but she had never accepted his lifestyle. He was coming to visit and either she would accept his lifestyle or she would never see him again. My mother told him, "John, you are my son and I love you with all of my heart. Nothing can ever change my love for you, but I cannot accept your lifestyle because it is biblically wrong." She said they stayed up most of the night talking about right and wrong, what the Bible says and about what true love really means. At one point, John said he didn't even believe there was a God.

My mother told me the hardest thing she ever did was to watch John as he got ready to board the plane, turn to give her one last chance to accept his lifestyle, then turn away knowing she may never see him again. She continued to pray for John's deliverance. It was three weeks before Christmas.

Three days before Christmas, God answered my mother's prayers in a miraculous way. You know the most familiar story of this type of transformation: Saul was on the road to Damascus when Jesus appeared to him (*Acts 9*). Saul was transformed from the inside out.... even his name was changed--to Paul. Yes, Paul, the one who wrote so many of the books in the New Testament. Everyone who has a true encounter with Jesus Christ is changed and transformed from the inside out.

John told me the story of God's visitation that night, three days before Christmas in 1985. He was getting ready for bed, looked at the clock, then turned off the light. All of a sudden, there was God! John said he didn't see God's face but His spirit filled the entire room and God's spirit consumed him. John said he "felt like trash and wanted to run away and hide but there was no place to go." How true, where can you run to escape God's presence? He knows all and He sees all. His spirit was upon John. Then God spoke, "John, I love you and I have a plan for your life if you will just love and trust me." When John shared this with me, I thought it was interesting that God did not go into all of the doctrinal issues we struggle with such as "be sprinkled" or "be totally immersed for baptism." You know, the things that really won't matter in *eternity* when you see God face to face.

Then God took John to heaven. John wasn't sure if he was actually in heaven or if it was a vision, but he cried out to God because he knew he didn't belong there. Instantly, John found himself back in his bed. He wanted to tell me so badly of the awesomeness of heaven but there were no words to describe the magnitude and the holiness of it. He just knew this was a place he wanted to live in for eternity but he knew he needed to be holy to live there.

For the next two hours, God showed John things from his past, things from his present, and things from his future. When God's presence finally lifted, John's bed was soaking wet from the tears he had cried. Time had passed so quickly, it seemed like a few moments instead of the two hours since he had last looked at his clock.

John didn't know what to do next. The following morning, he contacted the only Christian he knew at his work. He shared the story and was immediately told of the 'four steps' you must take to become a Christian. John joined him in the sinner's prayer and was told he was now a "Christian." I told John that if God's *miraculous* appearance before him didn't change his life, then he deserved to go to hell. Every Christian I know has accepted Christ by faith without any dramatic events, visions or visitations.

Baby Christian

I'm not sure why God appeared to John the way He did, but perhaps it was because He knew it was what John needed to come to Him and to trust Him. I do know that it was an act of amazing love, grace, and mercy on God's part. If we could truly fathom the deep love God has for each of us, we would never be defeated in our daily walk. I guess that is why it is called faith. *Hebrews 11:6 - And without faith it is impossible to please God, because anyone who comes to Him must believe that He exists and that He rewards those who earnestly seek Him.*

For the next six months, God talked with John on a daily basis, giving him instruction and performing many supernatural things in his life. I remember clearly the day God ceased speaking to him. John called me frantically crying, "God has left me. He's not talking to me anymore. What have I done to make Him leave? Am I going to hell now?" I explained to John that it was finally time for him to live his life in faith like the rest of us. God had supernaturally carried John for all of those months and now it was time for John to walk on his own.

You see, when we come to Christ, we are babes spiritually, and just like babies, we must learn to roll over, then crawl, then walk, then run. We may be old in our fleshly bodies, but our spirits need to grow and mature as we take in God's Word. Being a Christian is a lifelong process of continual growth. None of us will "arrive" until the day we see Him face to face.

Hebrews 5:12-14 NLT - You have been believers so long now that you ought to be teaching others. Instead, you need someone to teach you again the basic things about God's word. You are like babies who need milk and cannot eat solid food. For someone who lives on milk is still an infant and doesn't know how to do what is right. Solid food is for those who are mature, who through training have the skill to recognize the difference between right and wrong.

I loved John very much and was so grateful that God brought him back into our lives. Our family was unified through the working of God's Holy Spirit. When the family came together, we had one thing on our hearts and minds: the love and restoration God had brought into each of us. Our connection was deeper than it had ever been when we were growing up because the foundation was now the total epitome of love, Jesus Christ.

John's Passing

John was HIV positive for at least twenty-four years but did not contract full-blown AIDS until the end of his life. Those who he had been in contact with during those years of living a homosexual lifestyle had passed away many years earlier. God breathes life into our very being and it was God who kept John alive all of those years. The doctors were amazed at each checkup how John was able to live without a functioning immune system. Doctors wanted him to take the "drug cocktail" used today in HIV and AIDS treatment, but John chose to take only one drug, and live by faith in God's healing and sustaining power.

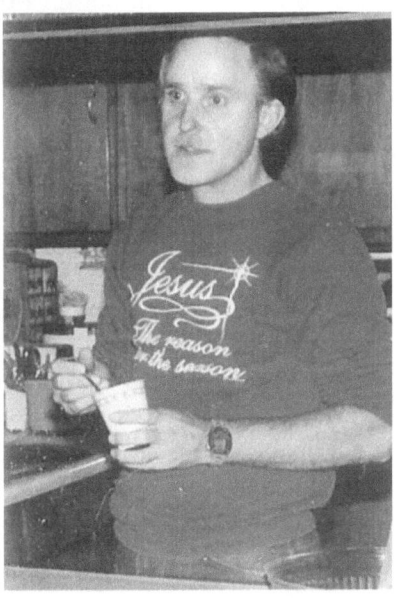

John loved this sweatshirt because of what it said.
Jesus - The reason for the season

John developed a brain tumor that caused the right side of his face to become paralyzed, as in Bells Palsy. This particular tumor usually takes years to affect the face in this way, but because John had no immune system, it happened within a couple of weeks. In the end, John was in the hospital only one week with the last couple of days being placed in hospice. He fell into a coma, lying motionless in the hospital bed. Our sister, Pam, and sister-in-law, Cleo, felt they should pray for him. They felt that John wanted permission to go home. During the prayer, they told him it was okay to leave to be with Jesus. He took one last breath, and then passed away peacefully. The amazing part of this story is that the tumor had no more power and his mouth was no longer paralyzed. He died with a smile on his face, proof that he was now finally home, content, and at perfect peace.

Here is an excerpt from John's will exactly as it was written because I believe it will help you understand the person John was when he was living.

John Turner's Last Will And Testament
August 20, 2003

I do not believe in nor do I desire that a traditional funeral be planned or held after my death. Instead, I wish to have my body cremated and the remains buried at the national cemetery in Clarksville, Indiana. Once my spirit has left my body to go be with the Lord, it is ridiculous for those who knew me to gather and gaze on a lifeless carcass, saying over and over, "Doesn't he look good?" My response is, "No, I look and AM very dead (at least to this world, but certainly not the next) and my spirit that animated and expressed itself through this body is no longer here."

I also request that should others wish to honor the life I shared with them, that instead of flowers, that any gifts and monies be given to a charitable organization that will benefit the LIVING...not the dead and departed. It is my request that the surviving family members and friends meet for a meal at the home of a family member… NOT an IMPERSONAL FUNERAL PARLOR, for the purpose of acknowledging how precious life is as it comes from the hand of God, and to reflect on the blessings of relationships as God purposed and planned it to be in setting up the institution of the FAMILY.

Do not be sad that I am now in Heaven with my Lord. Believe me, I would much rather be where I am than where you are, and I pray for the time when you will be here as well. I am now able to look directly into the face of the One Who paid such an awesome price to get me where I am. If anything, I will now have an eternity to jump and shout for joy that I "MADE IT!" simply because of the awesome grace and mercy of my Savior and Lord.

To the family or friends I leave behind that do not know Jesus as Lord, I beg you to let go of those things that are temporal and have little or no eternal value. If you face death without a Savior, you will never know the joy of living forever in this wonderful place but instead will be eternally separated from the Creator God Who made you for an awesome purpose and plan. Heaven is wonderful because Jesus is here. Don't miss it!!

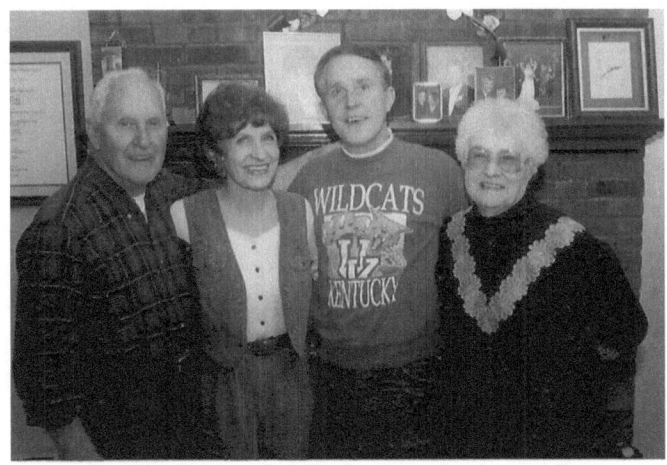

Here I am with Dad, John and Mom. They are rejoicing in heaven!

Keep Your Fork
Author Unknown

A young woman was diagnosed with a terminal illness and was given three months to live. As she was getting her things "in order," she contacted her pastor and had him come to her house to discuss certain aspects of her final wishes. She told him which songs she wanted sung at the service, what Scriptures she would like read, and what outfit she wanted to be buried in. Everything was in order and the pastor was preparing to leave when the young woman suddenly remembered something very important to her.

"There's one more thing," she said excitedly. "What's that?" came the pastor's reply. "This is very important," the young woman continued. "I want to be buried with a fork in my right hand." The pastor stood looking at the young woman, not knowing quite what to say. "That surprises you, doesn't it?" the young woman asked. "Well, to be honest, I'm puzzled by the request," said the pastor.

The young woman explained: "My grandmother once told me this story, and since then I have always tried to pass along its message to those I love and those who are in need of encouragement."

"In my years of attending socials and dinners, I always remember that when the dishes of the main course were being cleared, someone would inevitably lean over and say, "Keep your fork." "It was my favorite part because I knew that something better was coming, like velvety chocolate cake or deep-dish apple pie. Something wonderful, and with substance! So, I just want people to see me there in that casket with a fork in my hand and I want them to wonder, "What's with the fork?" Then I want you to tell them: "Keep your fork, the best is yet to come."

The pastor's eyes welled up with tears of joy as he hugged the young woman good-bye. He knew this would be one of the last times he would see her before her death, but he also knew that she had a better grasp of heaven than he did. In fact, she had a better grasp of what heaven would be like than many people twice her age, those with twice as much experience and knowledge. She knew something better was coming.

At the funeral, people were walking by the young woman's casket and saw the fork placed in her right hand. Over and over, the pastor heard the question, "What's with the fork?" And over and over again he smiled.

During his message, the pastor told the people of his conversation with the young woman shortly before she died and what the fork symbolized to her. He expressed how he could not stop thinking about the fork and how they probably would not stop thinking about it either. So the next time you reach down for your fork, let it remind you, that the best is yet to come!

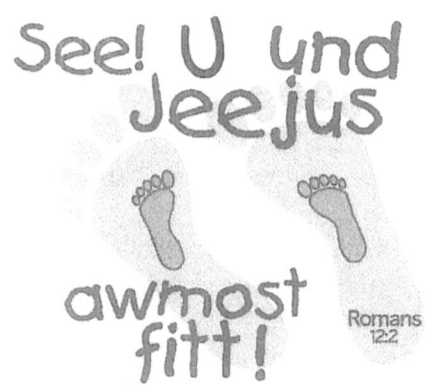

See! U und Jeejus awmost fitt! Romans 12:2

After John's experience with God, he began to see God differently. He was no longer GOD, but He was now Daddy God, John's loving heavenly Father. John started *Lytle Smyles*, which demonstrated how we as His children could view God from the eyes of a child!

Perhaps as you have read the story about John, you are thinking it seems too miraculous to be true. I can guarantee you it is, in fact, true. We serve a God of never-ending miracles, but now you must decide if *you* will believe. We live in a world where good and evil exist and there is a constant battle between the two for your soul.

Where you spend eternity is determined by one decision. What will you do with Jesus Christ, the One who came to pay the price on the cross that will save you from your sins? His blood will cover every sin you have committed so you can have a second chance on life. Your past will be washed away, never to be remembered anymore. How can you possibly pass up this amazing opportunity? I'm not saying it will be easy because we do have an enemy, but I can promise that it will be worth any price you have to pay, because He is still and has always been *"Lookin' At You, Kid!"*

Chapter Nine

Nuggets and Advice

It is vital that women perform breast self-examinations on a regular basis to find any suspicious lump or rash. Inflammatory breast cancer is a rare type of advanced breast cancer that appears like an infection on the skin with redness, warmth, and possibly swelling. If the rash does not clear up after two weeks of antibiotics, a biopsy of the underlying tissue should be performed. Survival rate for this aggressive breast cancer is about eighteen months.

Breast self exams were frustrating for me because of the fibrocystic disease. My breasts were full of lumps that kept moving so mammograms and ultrasounds were my screening for prevention. The tiny cluster of micro calcifications was found in my left breast and was barely detectable on the x-ray. The technician's trained eye could see the potential danger. The mammogram saved my life by finding the breast cancer at an early stage. Unless there is something suspicious, it is suggested that a woman have a mammogram once a year after the age of 40.

Selecting a surgeon to walk through this journey with you is crucial. You must have confidence not only in his ability to perform the surgery but also to listen to your concerns and answer questions so you understand clearly. Most women know their bodies. If you have a doctor who is not listening to your concerns, leave that doctor and find one who will take your concern seriously. Having someone with you at your doctor's appointment will help in hearing information you might miss as well as being there for support.

Most hospitals have a women's clinic to help those who are facing cancer. The staff members are knowledgeable registered nurses who can answer any questions. They encourage women to call with any concerns they may have, they offer support groups to help work through the process, they offer one-on-one education as well as educational classes, and have a lending library with material that covers a range of subjects to assist the patients, caregivers, and families during the cancer journey.

Cancer Services of Northeast Indiana is one of the best-kept secrets for those facing cancer. They offer the same services as the women's clinics in a hospital as well as transportation to and from chemotherapy and radiation treatments. Wigs, turbans, hats, scarves, bandages, and breast prostheses are provided at no cost. They also have a loan program of equipment for home recuperation such as hospital beds, shower benches, and wheelchairs.

The most amazing surprise for me about Cancer Services was finding that they offer financial assistance to those who qualify. They encourage submission of financial information because your financial situation would change if you had to take a leave of absence from your job, or had to quit due to your diagnosis. They qualify you according to where you are financially today rather than what you made last year. Check to see if your area may have an organization similar to Cancer Services.

What I've Learned

There were so many times I questioned why I had to go through so much for a simple stage one, no node involvement tumor, but what I have learned and the inner growth I have experienced from this six-year ordeal far outweighs the physical pain I experienced. Going through the pain is what brings true growth. Pearls are born out of the irritation from the tiny piece of sand. The oil flows only when the olive is crushed. I know God wants everything I go through to bring growth and to strengthen my character. *2 Chronicles 16:9 – For the eyes of the Lord range the earth to strengthen those whose hearts are fully committed to Him.*

The poem, The Weaver, meant so much to me during this time because it showed how God's plan is much bigger than what we can see.

THE WEAVER
Benjamin Franklin

My life is but a weaving
Between my Lord and me;
I cannot choose the colors
He worketh steadily.

Oft times He weaveth sorrow
And I, in foolish pride,
Forget He sees the upper,
And I the under side.

Not till the loom is silent
And the shuttles cease to fly,
Shall God unroll the canvas
And explain the reason why.

The dark threads are as needful
In the Weaver's skillful hand,
As the threads of gold and silver
In the pattern He has planned.

I have learned to make life-style changes such as watching what and how much I eat. Sugar and stress are two major factors in developing cancer. In fact, PET scans use radioactively labeled glucose to detect sugar-hungry tumor cells. Other changes I've made include taking supplements that help build my immune system, exercising more, and weeding out the things in my life that cause stress. I am still working on doing better with the exercise and stress!

I've learned to not sweat the small stuff. When I worry or get upset, it produces stress, which is not good for keeping my body disease-free. When you break down the word "disease," dis-ease, it literally means we are not at ease in our body, mind, and spirit. Studies have shown that 85% of all illness is stress related. In fact, the World Health Organization has proclaimed stress to be the number one global epidemic.

Stress Management
Author Unknown

A lecturer, when explaining stress management to an audience, raised a glass of water and asked, "How heavy is this glass of water?" Answers called out ranged from three ounces to six ounces. The lecturer replied, "The absolute weight doesn't matter. It depends on how long you try to hold it. If I hold it for a minute, that's not a problem. If I hold it for an hour, I'll have an ache in my right arm. If I hold it for a day, you'll have to call an ambulance. In each case, it's the same weight, but the longer I hold it, the heavier it becomes." He continued, "And that's the way it is with stress management. If we carry our burdens all the time, sooner or later, as the burden becomes increasingly heavy, we won't be able to carry on. As with the glass of water, you have to put it down for a while and rest before holding it again. When we're refreshed, we can carry on with the burden. So, before you return home tonight, put the burden of work down. Don't carry it home. You can pick it up tomorrow. Whatever burdens you're carrying now, let them down for a moment if you can. Relax; pick them up later after you've rested. Life is short. Enjoy it!"

And then he shared some ways of dealing with the burdens of life:

* Accept that some days you're the pigeon, and some days you're the statue.
* Always keep your words soft and sweet, just in case you have to eat them.
* Always read stuff that will make you look good if you die in the middle of it.
* Drive carefully. It's not only cars that can be recalled by their Maker.
* If you can't be kind, at least have the decency to be vague.
* If you lend someone $20 and never see that person again, it was probably worth it.
* It may be that your sole purpose in life is simply to serve as a warning to others.
* Never buy a car you can't push.
* Never put both feet in your mouth at the same time, because you won't have a leg to stand on.
* Nobody cares if you can't dance well. Just get up and dance.
* Since it's the early worm that gets eaten by the bird, sleep late.
* The second mouse gets the cheese.
* When everything's coming your way, you're in the wrong lane.
* Birthdays are good for you. The more you have, the longer you live.

* You may be only one person in the world, but you may also be the world to one person.
* Some mistakes are too much fun to only make once
* We could learn a lot from crayons. Some are sharp, some are pretty and some are dull. Some have weird names, and all are different colors, but they all have to live in the same box.
* A truly happy person is one who can enjoy the scenery on a detour.

There is a saying: *Worry is the dark room in which negatives can develop.* You need to stay positive and surround yourself with people who are positive, who believe, and who have faith for renewed strength on a daily basis. The words you speak are very powerful and can bring life or death. <u>Proverbs 18:21</u> - *The tongue has the power of life and death.* So speak LIFE!

This experience has helped me to be more patient. I try to not react immediately, to take a deep breath, and wait before saying anything. I try to leave the room so I don't say something I will regret. I ask myself the question, "In the light of eternity, does this really matter?"

I've learned to not take myself too seriously. A sense of humor is so important for maintaining sanity. Laughter is good medicine and it doesn't cost a thing! Patch Adams uses laughter therapy in his practice and it works very well. Laughter reduces stress, boosts your immune system, and it increases the oxygen in your body. We all know cancer cells are destroyed in the presence of oxygen. So help kill the cancer by laughing more! I love the saying: *We don't stop laughing because we grow old. We grow old because we stop laughing.*

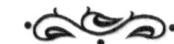

Healing Scriptures

I would love to share a list of healing Scriptures that I have taped to my bathroom mirror so I am reminded often of God's promises! Every morning I wake up and say out loud, "God, I thank You that You spoke this world into existence through Your Word and it's Your Word that I claim in my life today. 'Jesus was wounded for my transgressions and He was bruised for my iniquity, surely He bore my sorrows and by His stripes I am healed.' Your Word also says, 'I shall not die but live to declare the works of the Lord'."

Take a Scripture or two to declare over your life as you believe and receive God's promises. Make the promise personal by inserting your name or using "my" or "me" because these promises are for you direct from the throne of God.

Exodus 15:26 – *For I am the Lord who heals you.*

Exodus 23:25 – *Worship the Lord your God, and His blessing will be on your food and water. I will take away sickness from among you.*

Deuteronomy 7:15 – *The Lord will keep you free from every disease.*

Deuteronomy 30:19 – *I have set before you life and death, blessings and curses. Now choose life, so that you and your children may live.*

Psalm 30:2-3 NLT - *O Lord my God, I cried to you for help, and you restored my health. You brought me up from the grave. Oh, Lord, You kept me from falling into the pit of death. 5b – His favor lasts a lifetime! Weeping may last through the night, but joy comes with the morning.*

Psalm 30:11-12 NLT – *You have turned my mourning into joyful dancing. You have taken away my clothes of mourning and clothed me with joy, that I might sing praises to you and not be silent. O Lord my God, I will give you thanks forever!*

Psalm 33:18-19 NKJV – *Behold, the eye of the Lord is on those who fear Him, on those who hope in His mercy to deliver their soul from death, and to keep them alive in famine.*

Psalm 34:18-20 – *The Lord is close to the brokenhearted and saves those who are crushed in spirit. A righteous man may have many troubles, but the Lord delivers him from them all. He protects all his bones; not one of them will be broken.*

Psalm 37:39-40 KJV - *He is their strength in the time of trouble. And the Lord shall help them and deliver them.*

Psalm 40:17 NKJV- *I am poor and needy; yet the Lord thinks upon me. You are my help and my deliverer. Do NOT delay, oh my God.*

Psalm 41:1-3 NKJV – *The Lord will deliver him in time of trouble. The Lord will preserve him and keep him alive. The Lord will strengthen him on his bed of illness. You will sustain him on his sickbed.*

Psalm 103:1-5 – *Praise the Lord, all my inmost being, praise His holy name..... Who forgives all your sins, who heals all your diseases, who redeems your life from the pit, and crowns you with love and compassion, who satisfies your desires with good things, so that your youth is renewed like the eagles.*

Psalm 107:20 – *He sent forth His word and healed them, He rescued them from the grave.*

Psalm 107:41 *He lifted the needy out of their affliction.*

Psalm 118:17 NKJV – *I shall not die, but live and declare the works of the Lord.*

Proverbs 4:20-23 NKJV –*Incline your ear to my sayings do not let them depart from your eyes; keep them in the midst of your heart; for they are life to those who find them and health to all their flesh.*

Isaiah 53:5 NKJV - *He was wounded for our transgressions, He was bruised for our iniquities; the chastisement for our peace was upon Him, and by His stripes we are healed.*

Isaiah 54:17 NKJV – *No weapon formed against me shall prosper.*

Jeremiah 30:17 NKJV - *"For I will restore health to you and heal you of your wounds," says the Lord.*

Nahum 1:9 NKJV – *Affliction will not rise up a second time.*

Mark 16: 17-18 NKJV - *And these signs shall follow those who believe....they will lay hands on the sick and they will recover.*

John 15:7 KJV – *If you abide in me, and my words abide in you, you shall ask what you will and it shall be done unto you.*

Romans 8:11 - *And if the Spirit of Him who raised Jesus from the dead is living in you, He who raised Christ from the dead will also give life to your mortal bodies through His Spirit, who lives in you.*

II Corinthians 10:4-5 NKJV – *Casting down arguments and every high thing that exalts itself against the knowledge of God, bringing every thought into captivity to the obedience of Christ.*

Philippians 4:19 KJV – *But my God shall supply all my need according to His riches in glory by Christ Jesus.*

Hebrews 10:23 NKJV - *Let us hold fast the confession of our hope (faith), without wavering, for He who promised is faithful.*

III John 1:2 KJV - *Beloved, I wish above all things that thou mayest prosper and be in health, even as thy soul prospers.*

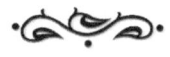

Butterflies

Butterflies have always meant a lot to me because of what they symbolize. If someone tries to help a butterfly escape from the cocoon, it will not be able to fly. The butterfly alone must complete the struggle in the cocoon so it will have the strength needed to fly. Here is an excerpt from my CD, "Change" and a poem written for me by a precious friend who knew of my love for butterflies.

Butterflies are beautiful and magnificent in design, each one unique in size, markings, and color. They were not always that way. Each begin as a caterpillar limited to crawling on the ground and in trees waiting for the day they will become what they were created to be.... a beautiful butterfly.

The metamorphosis from caterpillar to butterfly is not without struggle. The same holds true in our lives. Struggles and times of great trials actually strengthen us and take us to another level of faith and trust.

Though the cocoon binds tightly and we feel confusion, doubt, and despair, it symbolizes God's protection during our time of struggle. Only in the darkness of the cocoon can we be strengthened with wings that will enable us to fly to heights we could never have imagined. Only after our struggle can we truly experience the ecstasy of freedom and the sweet taste of victory.

Poem By Edie McKinney

Trapped in the darkness, waiting to grow
It's my time to change so I can let others know
The beauty of what I become is a leaf to unfold
For I feel God's touch and a story to be told

I am a willing vessel no longer trapped within my pain
I have given my heart to you Lord and now I have everything to gain
I soar above the treetops and let the wind catch my wings
My heart will be light and merry for a melody it sings

I can only be taken higher to a place somewhere in the sky
For I have been transformed into beauty and become that butterfly

Final Thoughts

Life takes many twists and turns. Many of those twists and turns may not be what we wanted or expected to happen in our lives. I know that I looked at life through 'rose-colored glasses' and expected only good things to happen. As naïve as that was, I see how the Lord continues to mold me into the woman of God that He desires for me to become. We need to guard our hearts and minds, as we stay focused on Him! Our heavenly Father keeps His loving and caring eyes on us because He has a plan!

Jeremiah 29:11- "For I know the plans I have for you," declares the LORD, "plans to prosper you and not to harm you, plans to give you hope and a future."

Malachi 3:3 – He will sit as a refiner and purifier of silver.

A silversmith must watch very carefully as he sits and holds a piece of silver in the middle of the fire where the flames are the hottest in order to burn away all of the impurities. If the silver is left a moment too long in the flames, it would be destroyed. The defining moment that the refining process is done is when the silversmith sees his image in the silver!

How very similar this is to our lives. God is forever watching over us as we face the most devastating of storms. God knows who you are, He knows where you've been, He knows your heart, and He knows what you are suffering through today. He allows us to be in the 'hottest' spot of the fire so the impurities in our lives will be burned away while keeping His eye on us at all times so that we will not be destroyed in the refining process. As we are pulled from the fire, what others see is His image shining through us.

If you have never made a commitment to Jesus Christ, I invite you to ask Him into your life as Savior and give Him complete control. You have tried living life your way. Why not try His? *Psalms 34:8 - Oh, taste and see that the LORD is good; blessed is the man who trusts in Him!* This one decision will change your life for eternity!

"Dear Lord Jesus, I am a sinner and know that I cannot save myself. I believe you died on the cross and rose again. I ask your forgiveness for my sins. Come into my heart and life and be my Savior. Thank you for saving my soul and giving me everlasting life. In Jesus Name I pray, AMEN!"

If you have said this prayer and believe upon Jesus Christ in your heart, you are now a part of the "family of God." Today is your spiritual birthday, but your spiritual *growth* is vital. Find a Bible-believing church for fellowship and accountability, read God's Word, The Holy Bible, and pray to your Father because He desires a relationship with you that is personal and intimate. God is no longer an 'entity' that lives out in the universe somewhere, but He is now your loving heavenly Father who lives in your heart through His Holy Spirit!

Never forget, *He's Lookin' At You, Kid!*

www.ingramcontent.com/pod-product-compliance
Lightning Source LLC
Chambersburg PA
CBHW030412290526
45785CB00004B/1975